Contents

List of Figures

Market-Based Demand Forecasting for Hospital Inpatient Services

James A. Rice and George H. Creel, II,
for the Society for Hospital Planning and Marketing
of the American Hospital Association

American Hospital Publishing, Inc.,
a wholly owned subsidiary
of the American Hospital Association

Library of Congress Cataloging in Publication Data

Rice, James A.
  Market-based demand forecasting for hospital inpatient services.

  Bibliography: p.
  1. Hospital utilization—Forecasting. I. Creel,
George H. II. Rossiter, Dean. III. Title. [DNLM:
1. Forecasting. 2. Health Services Research—
United States. 3. Hospital Planning—trends—
United States. WX 140 R496m]
RA971.3.R54 1984   362.1′1′0688   84-24265
ISBN 0-939450-26-7

Catalog no. 127124

© 1985 by
American Hospital Publishing, Inc.,
a wholly owned subsidiary of the
American Hospital Association

ᴀᴴᴬ is a service mark of American Hospital Association used under license by American Hospital Publishing, Inc.

Printed in the U.S.A.
2.5M-3/85-0079

Tamara Schiller, Editor
Peggy DuMais, Production
Marjorie Weissman, Manager, Book Editorial Department
Dorothy Saxner, Vice-President, Books

List of Tables

Preface

Most hospitals have recently initiated new or improved strategic planning and marketing processes. Unfortunately, the majority of these processes do not yet contain formal forecasting methods that quantify the expected demand for a hospital's several lines of business (for example, the number of admissions and patient days for cardiology customers in 1985). Hospital experience and literature are noticeably weak in the application of structured forecasting methods that reflect marketplace demographics and competitive forces. This book has been prepared in response to this void.

Introduction

Purpose of Book

This book has been developed by hospital planning and management practitioners to serve as a catalyst for hospital management and planners to:

- Pursue forecasting in a more structured and formal way than has occurred in the past
- Implement market-based demand planning techniques
- Focus on forecasting individual business unit demand (for example, orthopedics) instead of aggregate demand (for example, medical and surgical)
- Organize internal data sources to support market-based planning by linking diagnostic and financial data
- Assume a leadership role in encouraging all providers to make sound areawide data available
- Commit funds for refined forecasting models alone or in conjunction with neighboring hospitals

To achieve these goals, the book addresses hospital demand forecasting from a pragmatic management perspective, rather than an academic or theoretical perspective. As a result, the book does not focus on time series or other techniques rooted primarily in statistical theory, but on qualitative approaches that reflect the nature and characteristics of the health care marketplace.

1

Forecasting is often confused with planning. Hospital managers who say they would like a forecast often really mean they would like a plan to use as a guide to make something happen. This book is not about planning; it is about forecasting.

As an introduction to forecasting hospital inpatient demand, this book can be characterized as strategic more than operational, institutional more than departmental, and long range (five years) more than short range (next year).

It has been designed for use by hospital management and planning staff. Secondary audiences are students of hospital management, consultants, and areawide health systems planners.

The book is not a definitive treatise on the application of operations research techniques within hospital planning or marketing. Therefore, hospital managers need not be intimidated by the forecasting methods. In fact, a certain degree of irreverance and skepticism will be healthy as planning and marketing processes are strengthened from ideas in this book.

The authors have attempted to draw upon the contemporary thoughts and experiences of forecasters in other industries to develop applications for hospitals. However, continued refinements of these concepts are essential to improve the survivability of hospitals in an increasingly competitive environment.

For those who wish to move beyond the basics, selected citations and a bibliography of more sophisticated forecasting techniques, as well as more traditional statistical approaches, are included.

The book uses information from one hospital, Memorial Hospital, for examples of how to forecast specific services. Memorial is a 277-bed community hospital serving a growing suburban service area. It has an active and growing medical staff, and, until recently, its utilization had been growing since it opened in 1966. The hospital has been financially strong, but its management is now nervous about future utilization and financial status in an increasingly complex, uncertain, and competitive environment. For the first time, the hospital's management team is openly anxious about its ability to forecast the number and types of admissions, the number and types of outpatient and emergency department visits, and the work load of each of its several revenue centers. Management is uncomfortable basing projections on historical utilization trends that do not reflect future competition, regulation, medical advances, and changes in physicians' styles of practice. The managers are not sure how to address the following questions:

- How many admissions will each of our services have five years from now?
- How is our utilization likely to change as the population ages during the next 10 years?
- What would happen to utilization if we lost 10 percent of our market share in medical and surgical?
- What will our case mix be five years from now, and how will this affect our need for facility and staffing changes?
- What marketing objectives should we establish in our cardiology or oncology services?

Other hospitals may be experiencing the same concerns. This book is designed to help them develop market-based planning techniques to answer these questions more effectively and efficiently than with older methods. Major concepts and methods of hospital demand forecasting are presented by describing the experiences of a community hospital. These concepts and methods can be applied to hospitals varying from small, rural hospitals to large urban centers.

Reference is made to medical specialties throughout the book. Ideally, data will be available to enable DRG-specific forecasting. Hospitals should at least begin with specialty-focused forecasting, because data are more readily available and because management and marketing strategies will be directed at influencing demand by service or specialty rather than by diagnosis-related group (DRG).

Summary

This book is intended as an introduction to hospital demand forecasting. It does not seek to be a definitive treatise on elaborate operations research techniques. It seeks to stimulate more hospital managers and consultants to intensify their efforts in strengthening the quality of demand forecasting concepts, models, and data for U.S. community hospitals. In particular, much work is needed to improve forecasting demand for hospitals' outpatient and emergency service roles.

Much investment is needed. It is hoped that this book will encourage others to make such investments.

Chapter 1

Preparing for Demand Forecasting

Hospital managers who realize that their hospital must operate and compete in an increasingly complex and competitive environment will recognize that, in large part, their ability to survive, let alone thrive, in such an environment will be a function of the quality and accuracy of their decision-making processes. The application of various principles and practices of hospital demand forecasting can make a major contribution to the refinement of the manager's decision-making processes. To be better prepared to take advantage of the contributions that can accrue from strengthened demand forecasting, hospital managers must be individually prepared for the use of new forecasting approaches, prepare the organization to participate in the forecasting process, and encourage other members of the hospital management team to use the forecasts when making decisions. This chapter is intended to assist hospital management prepare itself for expanded use of forecasting techniques in the area of hospital demand. Strategic planning and marketing processes, the hospital manager's role, basic principles of forecasting, and information for a forecasting data base are discussed.

Role of Demand Forecasting in Strategic Planning and Marketing

Forecasting is concerned with determining what the future is apt to look like, rather than what it should look like, which is the job of planning.

The forecast provides input to the planning model. The forecasting model can be used to find out what the world will be like if it is left alone, if assumptions about the future are made, or if changes are made.

The forecasting process, therefore, plays an integral part in the important decision-making processes within hospitals. Although the processes hospital managers use to arrive at decisions vary with their background and style, certain basic elements are common to all decision making. Members of the hospital management team must take into account their knowledge of the existing situation and expectations of how the system and its components will change over time. This necessarily implies a forecast of what changes will take place and how the factors under consideration will be affected by these changes. If the historical trends and conditions for a hospital's emergency department market are projected statistically and the hospital introduces a new emergency service, two implied assumptions are that consumer preferences and care-seeking habits will not change and that new services will not be introduced by competing hospitals or medical clinics.

As the understanding of how things operate and the accuracy of forecasts improves, so will performance in planning and decision making, about both short-term and long-term situations. The more uncertain a hospital's management team is about the future, the more flexible and adaptive the hospital planning and marketing processes must be in order to cope with deviations from assumptions and estimates about the future.

Forecasting hospital demand contributes to a hospital's efforts to strengthen its strategic planning process by making available more explicit and more accurate information about the future, that is, the operating environment of the hospital and the implications of that environment on demand for the hospital's various services.

However, complex strategic planning models generally do not result in more accurate or acceptable plans for a hospital. In fact, the more complicated an institution's planning and forecasting processes are allowed to become and the more dependent it is upon only quantitative techniques, the more likely that the plans will not be understood or followed by decision makers within the hospital. Scott Armstrong, a forecasting author, states that managers should emphasize the value of simple forecasting methods. They are cheaper, easier to implement, and often more accurate than complex models. He also observes that, nevertheless, money continues to be invested in complex models. In responding to his self-posed question of why this is so, he states the following:

The rain dance has something for everyone. The dancer gets paid; the client gets to watch a good dance; the decision maker gets to shift the problem on to someone else in a socially acceptable way. (Who can blame him?) He hired the best dancer in the business. The major shortcoming of the rain dance is that it focuses the problem on something outside of us. The problem is due to the odds or to the environment—not to us. This attitude is more comfortable, but it is seldom valid in forecasting. Most problems in forecasting come from ourselves. For example: (1) we like to adjust to suit our biases, (2) we put too much faith in judgmental methods, (3) we fail to consider the relationship between the forecasting method and the situation, and (4) we confuse measurement models with forecasting models.*

Market-based hospital forecasting is also a relatively new refinement to decision-making processes in hospitals. Although the exact distinction between the decision-making processes of a hospital's planning and marketing is widely debated and contested, both perspectives are necessary to the ultimate vitality of the hospital organization.

At present, physicians are the principal customers of most of the hospital inpatient services. However, there is growing evidence that patients and their families are beginning to make significantly more independent decisions about which hospital to turn to and which services to use.

Hospital marketing is a structured process that identifies, evaluates, plans for, and manages exchange relationships between each of the hospital's unique services or programs and certain discrete consuming publics. The exchange involves the presumption that individuals give up something of value to the hospital in order to receive something of value in return. For example, patients give up money, time, convenience, power, or prestige for specific services that are judged to be of high quality and reasonably priced. The basic purpose of this structured process is to manage the exchange relationships in such a manner as to achieve more appropriate utilization of the hospital's resources.

Appropriate utilization of the hospital's resources may require changing the behavior or buying patterns not only of the hospital's customers, but also of the hospital itself in terms of the manner in which its services are made available to its publics. Marketing texts frequently refer to hospital behavior as being measured in terms of the *place* in

---

*Armstrong, John Scott. *Long Range Forecasting: From Crystal Ball to Computer*, New York: John Wiley and Sons, 1978, page 399.

which services are made available, the *price* of these services (not just dollars, but time and convenience, as well), and the alternate forms of *packaging* and *promoting* the services. Forecasting hospital demand cannot be completed unless there is an understanding of how purchasing practices of physicians or patients may change in the future. Competition from other hospitals and medical clinics also influences the ultimate accuracy of the hospital's demand forecasts because of the importance these factors have in the share of discrete markets. Therefore, hospital demand forecasting must have a clear understanding of marketing factors that will influence the competitive posture of the hospital in all lines of business, as well as the receptivity of the various publics to using the services.

The structured techniques of hospital forecasting can also influence a hospital's development of marketing strategies. The use of "what-if" modeling techniques facilitates understanding and more rapid testing of the consequences of planning and marketing decisions. Hospital demand forecasting, therefore, plays an important interactive role within the hospital's planning and marketing decision-making processes: it not only is influenced by the implications of decisions that result from these processes, but also influences the scope and nature of management decisions.

Role of Management in Creating a Positive Organizational Climate

Hospital managers must recognize that a major commitment is required when establishing an organizational climate conducive to structured demand forecasting. Their level of understanding, skills, and proper attitude with respect to the need for and nature of forecasting efforts must be developed. In addition, the board of directors must understand that future demand is the function of many external forces over which they have little direct control, but that can dramatically influence the demand for services. The board members, as well as department managers, must participate in monitoring these factors and in judging their potential impact on the hospital's ultimate demand profile.

Hospitals must also be prepared to invest money in the development of staff and the procurement and maintenance of data necessary for hospital demand forecasting. This commitment of resources and energy cannot be a one-time or sporadic effort. The forecasting process must be an ongoing, integral element of the organization's strategic planning and marketing activities. The forecasts themselves are not as valuable as the process that decision makers move through to establish the forecasts and to evaluate the implication of these alternative demand forecasts on hospital operations.

Basic Principles of Forecasting

Although many useful forecasting techniques are available, the accuracy of forecasts ultimately depends on the skill of the forecasters in using available resources. As forecasting is more of an art than a science, there is no single method for ensuring that mistakes will not be made in forecasting a hospital's demand. However, by applying the following principles, it should be possible at least to avoid blunders or large-scale mistakes that lead to disastrous results.

In their efforts to establish a positive environment for improved forecasting, hospital managers can also take advantage of, or recognize and shape, the commitment to forecasting by considering the following basic forecasting principles.*

Formulating the problem. If the forecasting problem is to be properly formulated, several questions must be asked and answered: How is the demand forecast to be used? What decision will be based on the forecast, and when must this decision be made? What are the important factors in the hospital's delivery system, and how are they related to one another? What is the value of historical hospital demand information? Has the delivery system changed to such an extent that the historical information is irrelevant, or will an analysis of past data assist in understanding the existing system's operation? Have there been related hospital services that will offer insight into what might happen to a new program's implementation? Is good historical information available, or will it be costly to obtain?

Involving top management. Users of the research must be involved in the analytical process. This point is the key in forecasting hospital demand. Unless the appropriate managers participate actively in the forecasting process, there is little chance that they will use the forecast with any degree of confidence. In addition, they may consider it only superficially in their decision-making activities.

Choosing techniques. Because more than one technique is frequently used for a particular forecasting problem, the ability to identify which techniques to use and how to combine them depends on the skill of the forecaster. The forecaster should be problem-oriented rather than technique-oriented in order to serve the needs of decision makers effectively.

---

*Armstrong, John Scott. *Long Range Forecasting: From Crystal Ball to Computer*, New York: John Wiley and Sons, 1978.

Most industries have found that an eclectic approach to forecasting proves to be the most accurate and cost-effective. Forecasting hospital demand, therefore, benefits from the application of a variety of quantitative and judgmental techniques.

Knowing the current position. In order to estimate the future position of a boat or an automobile at a particular time, it is necessary to know the current speed of the vehicle, the rate at which its speed is changing, and its direction. Experience in other industries has shown that, unless thorough analysis of historical data is made, the changes in current market share rate or utilization rates may not be accurately known. No matter how significant the recent changes in the system have been, experience also shows that previous trends should not be discarded immediately. Although hospital demand forecasters must continually anticipate basic shifts in the underlying assumptions upon which hospitals' demand forecasts are generated, they cannot afford to ignore the past interaction of external factors on basic utilization experiences.

Measuring accuracy. Unless an analytical approach is used, a measure of the forecasting error or the accuracy of the forecast is very difficult to obtain. Accuracy is expressed in terms of a range, that is, with the assumption that the true value will fall within this range. Most features of hospital demand preclude the rigorous application of statistical probabilities. However, management should at least attempt to achieve a group consensus on the probability of an event occurring or the specific impact the event will have on hospital demand.

Tracking the forecast. Revisions and updates are unlikely to be accomplished unless a formal system is set for collecting information and tracking the accuracy of the forecasts. The initial demand forecast may have been reasonable on the basis of information available at the time, but a comparison must be made of what is happening now and what was forecasted then to determine whether the earlier decisions should be revised.

Developing a sound data base. The establishment of improved demand forecasting methods in the hospital will, in large part, be a function of the scope, quality, and accessibility of data and of the hospital's existing operations and its relative position within the marketplace. Hospital managers must devote considerable time, energy, and resources to establishing and maintaining a data base for planning and forecasting that encompasses internal operating data, as well as external market information. Three basic caveats should guide hospital managers in their investment in the development and ongoing maintenance of this data base:

1. Demand forecasting is only as good as the data from which the forecasts are derived and the rigor with which judgments about the trends of the data are tempered. Although most hospitals will start with specialty-specific data, all must be prepared to use DRG-oriented data files for the future.
2. Quantitative methods can be applied to historical utilization information about all of the hospital's programs and their relative market share. These quantitative methods need not necessarily be complicated. The basic challenge is to meet the need for data, as well as to determine how to merge, store, sort, analyze, and interpret the data for planning.
3. The principal data required for improved forecasting are not alien to hospital managers; this same information is talked about and used every month during routine operations. The data include utilization statistics by each DRG, service, or department; demographic profiles on individuals residing within the service area; and market share measured by an evaluation of patient origin data from hospitals serving the same market area. The new challenge for hospital managers during the 1980s, however, is to:
   - Assemble and use cross-sectional analyses to examine these data elements in smaller, more discrete units than generally were used in the past
   - Evaluate the demographic profile of the service area, by discrete age and sex cohorts, in smaller geopolitical units than were employed in the past
   - Use demand forecasts by diagnosis or specialty rather than by aggregated services
   - Examine market share for all of the hospital's programs, services, or lines of business within discrete population groups and geopolitical market areas

The ability to conduct an analysis of existing data in these refined units will occur only as hospitals begin to merge their two principal data bases. These data bases are the abstract of clinical data associated with patient discharges, frequently submitted to local peer review organizations (PROs) or to abstracting services, and the hospital's financial records generally identified in billing records. The critical link between the two data files is the ability to match units of data for a specific patient's discharge.

The merged data base, once developed, must be maintained and updated. At first, the data base will be less accurate and more general than hospital managers will want to use in their forecasting and ultimately in their strategic planning and marketing activities. Medical record information and billing data files must be integrated, if not on an ongoing basis, at least once a year by sampling. Pressures will exist in the future for expansion of electronic data-processing applications in forecasting to handle the mass of hospital clinical and financial data. Additional creativity will be needed to procure data on the operations of competitors and on diverse publics.

Establishing data on the hospital's operating environment is dependent on the willingness of other hospital leaders to exchange patient origin and utilization statistics. These data must be organized by geopolitical unit and by specialty for all hospitals serving a market area.

Hospital managers will also need to invest in a variety of market research techniques to continually monitor the public's attitudes and opinions about each of the hospital's lines of business. This incorporation of trend analysis, consumer behavior and attitude profiles, and changing competitive environment will represent major challenges for hospital managers in the future. The ultimate effectiveness of forecasting, however, will be critically linked to the establishment of a data base that incorporates more detailed, more accurate, and more timely data on the external environment, as well as the internal operating experiences of the hospital and its several programs.

Chapter 2

Better Understanding of Hospital Demand Forecasting

Understanding demand for hospitals' services is becoming considerably more complex than it was during the 1970s. Hospitals are diversifying, no longer just providing treatment of acute illness but delivering a wide range of health services. Forecasting the demand for these various programs and services, therefore, has become a complex challenge. It is important to understand the nature of hospital demand and the factors that interact, causing future increases or decreases.

In general, hospitals are involved in four basic lines of business: inpatient services, outpatient services, ancillary services of a diagnostic or therapeutic nature, and subsidiary businesses that may or may not be related to patient care (see figure 1). Strategies for forecasting demand discussed in this book therefore focus on admissions and patient days, by specialty or program; emergency department and outpatient clinic visits, by service or program; and ancillary department work-load units as a function of demand for inpatient and outpatient services, for example, surgical procedures, laboratory tests, x-ray procedures, pharmacy prescriptions, and various therapy procedures. These strategies will strengthen hospitals' capabilities to forecast demand (utilization) for their traditional services and other major lines of business.

Historically, the health care industry has had an orientation to more demand and bigger facilities as a result of having few debt capacity constraints, little effective competition, and relatively minor regulatory infringements until the 1970s. However, these reasons are now of little

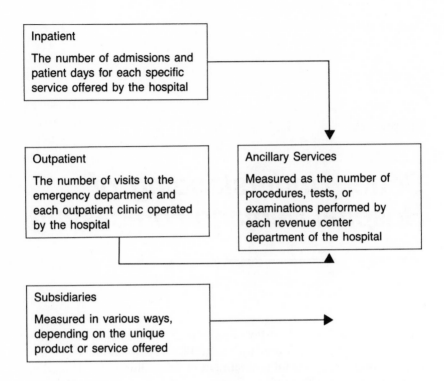

Figure 1 Utilization by line of business

consolation to the hospital manager attempting to forecast the demand for each business unit within each of several diverse lines of business.

Therefore, hospital planning has been preoccupied with facility planning and department budgeting. It was not until the late 1970s that government intervention, coupled with excess bed capacity in many cities, changed the nature of hospital planning. At present, five major environmental pressures necessitate refined demand and revenue forecasting techniques. These environmental pressures are demographic shifts, reimbursement shifts, scarcity of capital resources, competition for patients, and changing advances in medical technology.

Demographic Shifts

The U.S. population is growing at a moderate rate, but is aging rapidly. Although the post-World War II baby-boom generation is largely responsible for the increase in median age, the elderly are the fastest growing segment of the population (see figure 2). Such shifts in population demographics are significant to hospital managers inasmuch as the utilization of hospital services varies dramatically by age and sex (see table 1). Of all demographic characteristics (age, income level, race, urban-rural, sex, and so forth), age is the most important factor, then sex.

However, regional economics coupled with population migration can reinforce or reverse these national population trends at the local level. For example, the percentage of the population represented by the elderly varies from state to state. Hospital staff should recognize the importance of tracking the changes in both the size and composition of the service-

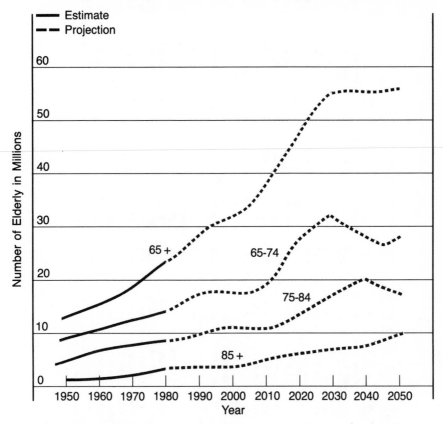

These data represent the entire census-level legal population. They do not include any data from the 1980 census.

Source: U.S. Bureau of the Census

Figure 2 Number of elderly in the United States, by age groups, 1950 to 2050

Table 1 Variable Hospital Use Rates for the United States, 1972 to 1976

Age/Sex Group	1976			1974			1972			% Change, 1972 to 1976		
	Admissions per 1,000	ALOS*	Patient Days per 1,000	Admissions per 1,000	ALOS*	Patient Days per 1,000	Admissions per 1,000	ALOS*	Patient Days per 1,000	Admissions per 1,000	ALOS*	Patient Days per 1,000
All Admissions	163.2	7.57	1,235.424	159.2	7.74	1,232.208	154.9	7.75	1,200.475	5.4	(2.3)	2.9
All Males	135.3	8.08	1,093.224	131.1	8.31	1,089.441	127.8	8.28	1,058.184	5.9	(2.4)	3.3
0-1	232.9	5.94	1,383.426	215.8	6.2	1,337.96	247.5	5.99	1,482.525	(5.9)	(.8)	(7.1)
1-4	101.5	3.93	398.895	99.4	4.34	431.396	101.2	4.25	430.1	.3	(.8)	(7.3)
5-14	58.5	4.15	242.775	60.8	4.4	267.52	60.5	4.27	258.335	(3.3)	(2.8)	(6.0)
15-24	79.8	5.9	470.82	78.7	6.21	488.727	75.9	6.01	456.159	5.1	(1.8)	3.2
25-34	92	6.5	598	91.4	6.82	623.348	88.5	6.69	592.065	4	(2.8)	1
35-44	121.7	7.3	888.41	118.8	7.69	913.572	119.1	7.5	893.25	2.2	(2.7)	(.5)
45-54	160.8	8.33	1,339.464	152.3	8.61	1,311.303	146.3	8.57	1,253.791	9.9	(2.8)	6.8
55-64	224.8	9.28	2,086.144	219.9	9.8	2,155.02	208.4	10.13	2,111.092	7.9	(8.4)	(1.2)
65-74	331.6	10.87	3,604.492	320.2	11.11	3,557.422	318.2	11.48	3,652.936	4.2	(5.3)	(1.3)
75+	503.4	11.95	6,015.63	474.1	12.05	5,712.905	441.8	12.17	5,376.706	13.9	(1.8)	11.9
All Females	189.2	7.24	1,369.808	185.2	7.37	1,364.924	179.7	7.4	1,329.78	5.3	(2.2)	3
0-1	176.1	6.2	1,091.82	167.4	6.24	1,044.576	184.2	5.82	1,072.044	(4.4)	6.5	1.8
1-4	78.8	3.86	304.168	77.1	4.04	311.484	77.3	4.16	321.568	1.9	(7.2)	(5.4)
5-14	49.9	4.35	217.065	51.8	4.25	220.15	51.1	3.96	202.356	(2.3)	9.8	7.3
15-24	199.7	4.32	862.704	205.3	4.39	901.267	214.1	4.46	954.886	(6.7)	(3.1)	(9.7)
25-34	241.9	5.03	1,216.757	244	5.16	1,259.04	247.2	5.18	1,280.496	(2.1)	(2.9)	(5.0)
35-44	181.9	6.56	1,193.264	188.9	7.11	1,343.079	184.2	6.95	1,280.19	(1.2)	(5.6)	(6.8)
45-54	191.8	7.96	1,526.728	189.6	8.12	1,539.552	179.5	8.39	1,506.005	6.9	(5.1)	1.4
55-64	209.6	9.6	2,012.16	197.1	9.74	1,919.754	180.4	10.06	1,814.824	16.2	(4.6)	10.9
65-74	274	11.04	3,024.96	268.1	11.39	3,053.659	260.8	11.85	3,090.48	5.1	(6.8)	(2.1)
75+	456.1	12.11	5,523.371	423.5	12.91	5,467.385	392.7	13.45	5,281.815	16.1	(10)	4.6

Source: U.S. Department of Health, Education, and Welfare, National Health Survey, series 13, numbers 19, 26, and 37

*ALOS = average length of stay

area population. Although total population is important, the crucial element for market-based planning is the age-sex distribution, which affects not only the amount of demand for inpatient lines of business, but also the type of service (see figure 3).

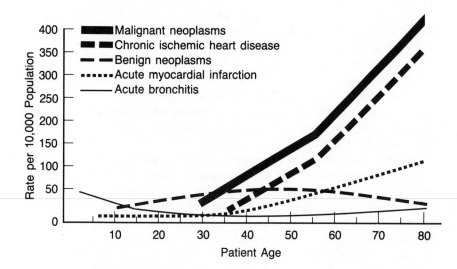

Sources: National Center for Health Statistics and The Hospital Research and Educational Trust, Chicago

Figure 3 Admission rates for selected diagnostic conditions

There are dramatic differences in use rates (admissions or patient days per thousand population) and average length of stay (ALOS) among age and sex cohorts (a group having statistical factors in common) (see table 1). The ALOS for patients older than 75 is about twice that of patients aged 25 to 34. Similarly, the patient-day use rate for males older than 75 is ten times the rate for the 25- to 34-year cohort and, for females, more than four times as great. Differences among the sexes, although not as wide, are significant. This information focuses attention on the need for demand forecasting techniques to incorporate population demographics and use rates explicitly.

Variability in demand also exists between men and women of different age groups for each business unit. Each age-sex cohort will experience different demands for surgical interventions. Forecasts of future demand, therefore, should take into consideration expected changes in the age and sex profiles of a hospital's market area. Managers should be prepared to monitor and predict these demographic shifts or run the risk of overestimating or underestimating the expected utilization (demand) for the hospital's different inpatient services.

Hospital Payment Shifts

As a result of recent concerns about public expenditures for health, three basic trends can be identified in hospital financial management:
- More prospective payment
- More payment by case mix or DRGs
- More aggressive rate review at the service or department level, as well as at the aggregate hospital level

These payment shifts will require stronger demand forecasting. The shift to prospective payment will require hospital managers to know their future revenue needs more accurately. This will, in turn, place the hospital in a precarious negotiating posture with third-party payers if expected demand and corresponding resource requirements are not known in advance. In addition, the hospital will be at substantial financial risk if the forecasted amount is not actually received. Because revenue is a function of units of services used (demanded) and the average charge per unit, faulty forecasts of demand, perhaps even more than improper pricing, will jeopardize the institution's future financial viability.

The shift to reimbursement on a case-mix or DRG basis further exacerbates the critical nature of forecasts for units of service used. Not only must the number of aggregate units be accurately forecasted, but the types of units also become crucial.

There is a dramatic variation in revenue associated with the many lines of business in a general community hospital (see table 2). An average oncology admission can produce approximately $3,000 of revenue, whereas a pediatric admission represents only approximately $750 of revenue. If a hospital were being paid on an average case-mix profile that assumed several oncology and relatively few pediatric admissions, the hospital would have substantial gross revenues available to offset its operating costs. If actual experience during the fiscal year yielded more pediatric admissions than oncology admissions, financial viability would be enhanced. However, if fewer oncology patients were admitted, financial disaster could result. Hospital demand forecasting should, therefore, become more accurate on a business unit basis, as well as on the aggregate hospital utilization.

In the past, the rate review bodies have focused much of their attention on aggregate per diem charges and have allowed hospital managers to shift surplus revenues from over-producing departments to cover shortfalls in other revenue centers. This financial flexibility may not be

Table 2 Relative Revenue Dependence upon Alternate Specialties
for a Suburban Community Hospital

Strategic Business Units, Ranked by Total Revenue		Revenue		
		Total (millions)	Percent of Total Hospital	Per Stay, $
1	General surgery	4.760	21.4	2,091
2	General medicine	2.744	12.3	1,407
3	Psychiatry	2.448	11.0	4,039
4	Chemical dependence	2.445	11.0	3,627
5	Orthopedic	2.261	10.2	2,041
6	Oncology	1.461	6.6	2,888
7	Cardiology	1.230	5.5	2,371
8	Obstetrics	1.225	5.5	846
9	Urology	1.005	4.5	1,801
10	Pediatrics	.735	3.3	752
11	Gynecology	.728	3.3	1,463
12	Neurology	.502	2.2	2,414
13	Otorhinolaryngology	.315	1.4	852
14	Ophthalmology	.282	1.3	1,438
15	Oral surgery	.123	.5	1,401
	Total	22.264	100.0	

available in the future. As rate review bodies probe to review specific
department and service charges, hospital managers will need to be more
accurate in setting charges, and, therefore, more accurate in forecasting expected revenues and expenses by department. These forecasts will
be only as good as the forecasts of the units of service expected
(demanded) for each ancillary department.

Hospital demand forecasting must become more accurate, not only
on an aggregate basis or by service, but within all revenue centers, particularly the heavy net revenue-producing diagnostic services areas. Forecasts of ancillary department work loads should be developed
recognizing the dramatic variability of procedures or tests per average
admission among departments, and the dramatic variability of demand
ratios among diagnostic-related admissions (see table 3).

Capital Resources

It is now almost axiomatic that hospitals have limited capital resources
to meet their complex community service roles. Competition for capital
is expected to intensify for the following critical reasons:

Table 3 Ancillary Revenue for Specialty Services

| Strategic Business Unit | Revenue Contribution per Day | | | | |
| | Room and Board | | Ancillary | | |
	$	%	$	%	Total $
Medical	148.90	49.6	151.19	50.4	300.09
Progressive cardiac	197.68	45.1	241.11	54.9	438.79
Surgical	148.38	34.4	283.22	65.6	431.60
Orthopedic	148.40	39.3	229.06	60.7	377.46
Chemical dependency	119.65	67.7	56.96	32.3	176.61
Pediatrics	152.77	42.4	207.92	57.6	360.69
Intensive care	386.02	41.8	537.91	58.2	923.93
Adolescent mental health	172.00	71.7	67.78	28.3	239.78
Mental health	155.56	73.6	55.82	26.4	211.38
Obstetrics	147.98	43.8	189.58	56.2	337.56
Nursery	87.73	66.5	44.19	33.5	131.92
Total	154.66	47.9	168.40	52.1	323.06

Source: Memorial Hospital billing records, FY 1981

- Capital funds are less available to health care as a result of capital requirements in other industries.
- Hospitals have eroded their equity base (ability to generate income plus contributions) as a result of Medicare requirements to spend depreciation funds or lose reimbursement of interest.
- Hospitals' need for capital, for example, the need to replace out-moded facilities and the need for working capital for diversification, are accelerating as the pace of technology changes.
- The volatility of hospital payments, weak financial performance of hospitals, and potential loss of the "franchise protection" provided by certificate-of-need legislation have made investors in tax-exempt bonds unsure about the security of their investment.

Hospitals' survival depends upon their ability to secure resources that are the correct amount, the correct type, available at the right time and place, and available at minimum cost. As a result of these factors, institutions that protect their access to capital in the competitive environment eventually will control the institutions that do not maintain their ability to access capital markets.

Managers' abilities to meet these capital formation challenges are linked to the accuracy of service demand forecasts. The hospital that can accurately forecast a shift in its service role to more outpatient primary care services will be better prepared to recruit, relocate, and reorient the proper number and type of personnel. Better forecasting, then, not only ensures that scarce capital is secured at more favorable terms, but also helps discern whether the hospital can secure the capital at all. Sound forecasting models provide greater lead time for management to plan for such resource requirements. In addition, an accurate assessment of activity levels allows hospitals to staff at an efficient level or to divest unprofitable activities.

Forecasting hospital demand should play an integral part in resource procurement and resource allocation decisions. Demand forecasting should be more timely, as well as more accurate, in order to maximize hospitals' capabilities to control and influence their future vitality in an era of scarce capital resources.

Competition

Hospitals will experience intensified competition for scarce financial resources and also greater competition. This competition is a challenge made increasingly complex by the following factors:

- Because some lines of business have stagnant or declining markets (for example, pediatrics), an increase in market share or market base may be necessary to remain in this line of business.
- Traditional competitors (other hospitals) are becoming smarter and more aggressive in their marketing practices, making it more difficult to maintain, let alone expand, market share to traditional lines of business.
- Preferred provider organizations and business coalitions are emerging and may play an influential role when employees of participating firms select a hospital. These organizations merit special attention, as they represent large blocks of charge-based patients; if possible, they will modify their employees' health care services consumption through differential pricing or coverage.
- As one of the largest industries at approximately 10 percent of the gross national product, the health care field will attract new competition from entrepreneurs outside the industry. Proprietary firms will take advantage of their ability to access capital markets and develop economies of scale.
- Hospital initiatives to diversify vertically or horizontally into non-traditional lines of business will create competitive pressure from

new competitors. Hospitals are rushing to provide such services as more ambulatory and geriatric care and chemical dependency treatment. These strategies can create tensions with practicing physicians, nursing homes, public health nursing organizations, and nonmedical treatment centers.

These factors combine to create an extremely dynamic and competitive health care marketplace that can no longer be ignored in demand forecasting. Techniques that incorporate explicit indicators of competition instead of implicit assumptions about historic trends should be adopted.

Technology Advances

Hospital demand is influenced in two ways by changes in medical technology. First, advances in diagnosis and treatment procedures tend to result in lower average lengths of stay, as well as in more procedures that can be performed safely on an outpatient basis (for example, fewer admissions for certain surgical procedures or diagnostic work-ups). Second, increased accuracy of diagnostic capabilities stimulates physicians to seek greater accuracy in their treatment via more intense use of more complex diagnostic procedures. The result of these two factors is that there are fewer admissions per thousand persons, but the potential for ancillary services on a per-admission or per-day basis is greater.

Forecasting ancillary department service demands, therefore, should be sensitive to changes in medical technology. The rapid pace of the changing character of this technology represents an additional motivation for hospital managers to develop and use new forms of forecasting models.

The continued significance of these five demand-influencing forces places intense pressure upon hospital managers to become more structured and sophisticated in the forecasting of service demands. There are not only more variables to be considered in forecasting service demand, but the amount and speed of interaction among these variables are becoming frustratingly more complex. Simple straight-line extrapolations of past experiences are not sufficient for hospital managers of the 1980s. The challenge is not only central to hospitals' future vitality, but also their viability.

Although the need for better forecasting systems has never been more pressing and timely, as an industry, the health care field can take some solace knowing that most hospitals are strengthening their strategic planning and marketing systems, reaching a high level of sophistication to accommodate new forecasting methods.* In addition, many hospitals are designating individuals (and in some cases, entire departments) to deal with forecasting, and advances in computer software and equipment enable hospital managers to handle more efficiently the volume of data and variety of manipulations required by the forecasting challenges of the 1980s.

The remaining chapters of this book are designed to assist hospital managers to take advantage of these developments by becoming more familiar with the practice of demand forecasting.

---

*See study results from Survey of Planning Practices in U.S. Hospitals, 1981, conducted by the Society for Hospital Planning of the American Hospital Association.

Chapter 3

The Demand Forecasting Process: Developing the Base-Case Forecast

The base-case forecast is only a *preliminary* definition of the hospital's expected demand; it provides a *base* for further planning, marketing, and forecasting. In general, the base case assumes that all demand-influencing factors, except the demographic profile of the service area, will remain unchanged in the future. The base case defines the parameters for subsequent steps in a hospital's planning and market-ing studies, as well as tests the reasonableness of assertions that the board, managers, or medical staff might make about future need for specific services. Although developing this initial forecast is a critical component in a hospital's overall planning and marketing processes, the base case is only a starting point. It is rarely an accurate prediction of actual future demand. Modification occurs as managers develop a better understanding of trends underlying the assumptions of the base case (see chapter 4).

Forecasting demand of a hospital's inpatient services requires a nine-stage process:
1. Defining service or market area
2. Forecasting market population profiles
3. Forecasting use rates by service or DRG
4. Forecasting aggregate demand for each service or DRG
5. Forecasting market share for each customer group

6. Forecasting the hospital's customer utilization for each service in terms of admissions and visits
7. Forecasting ALOS for each inpatient service
8. Forecasting patient days used for each inpatient service
9. Forecasting ancillary department work-load volumes

Hospitals can implement such a forecasting model either manually or by using computer software programs. Use of a computer to support such forecasting processes is not essential, but is increasingly desirable because of the large number of calculations required.

The logic behind the market-based forecasting model is not complex; however, the quantity of data can be large, and the quality of data can be poor. Subsequent sections of this book discuss not only the type and amount of data needed, but also essential elements of the path that guides the use of data to yield a reliable forecast of future demand.

This chapter describes the efforts of Memorial Hospital, a 277-bed suburban community hospital, to forecast the demand of its several services and departments. This case study moves through a step-by-step process of generating a base case for expected demand for several lines of business.

The case study will be used to illustrate the following four features of the process:

- Definitions: A description of concepts, their importance to hospital management, and basic definitions.
- Process: How to do the forecasting process in a step-by-step manner; samples of work sheets and checklists are provided.
- Issues: Practical factors to consider in moving through the steps.
- Data: Sources of data to use in the process.

Stage 1. Defining Service or Market Area

Definitions

A community hospital's service or market area can be defined as the geographic area in which the hospital intends to focus its resources and strategies in the foreseeable future. The region is the area in which the hospital will attempt to be recognized as a major provider of inpatient and outpatient services, or the geographic area within which the hospital has the responsibility for meeting the diverse service needs of persons living and working within it. As hospitals move into a new competitive era, this service area also can be viewed as where the hospital intends to maximize its market share, the area where the majority of persons who utilize inpatient and outpatient services will use the hospital, rather than other providers, for these services. Service areas can vary for different lines of business.

Process

The determination of historical service or market areas can be determined by a structured evaluation of the hospital's past *dependency rate.* The dependency rate represents the degree to which the hospital relies on certain communities for its various utilization volumes. In general, data to define historical dependency rates are obtained from the medical record department. Information of patient origin is collected by service, specialty, or DRG for each community and/or zip code.

It will become increasingly important for hospitals to know exactly from which area their customers are admitted, by community or census tract, as well as by zip code and, therefore, to have the ability to define their past and expected utilization by both of these categories. An understanding of dependency on zip code will be important as hospitals target direct-mail campaigns to specific segments of their service area. In addition, an understanding of community and census-tract origins for customers will become important as historical utilization is linked with historical population information. Population data are usually available only on a community or census-tract basis (see appendix A).

Using information from the medical record department or from various discharge abstracting sources, hospitals have three ways to define their principal service or market area:

Option 1. Traditionally, the geographic area that represents approximately 80 percent to 85 percent of inpatient admissions is the *principal market area* or *primary service area.* This definition will prove to be increasingly inadequate inasmuch as it deals only with aggregate admissions or discharge information. Ultimately, hospitals will need to define market areas for each line of business, for example, the market area for obstetrical activity, the unique geographic area for surgical patients, and the unique service area for mental health patients. Each line of business can have a distinctly different market area.

Option 2. The area that represents more than 2 percent of inpatient demand is the service area. For example, the primary service area would include all those communities that contribute at least 2 percent of the hospital's overall admissions or at least 2 percent of admissions by each line of business.

Option 3. The principal marketing area is that area in which the hospital has at least a 10 percent share of the market. For example, those communities or zip codes in which a hospital is responding to at least 10 percent of the actual demand (in aggregate or for each specific service) generated by residents would be part of the hospital's principal service area.

Memorial Hospital uses option 3. Seven communities and adjacent townships from three counties represent approximately 85 percent of Memorial's total admissions. This area also includes all communities in which Memorial provides 10 percent of the patient days and admissions utilized by that population (see table 4 and figure 4).

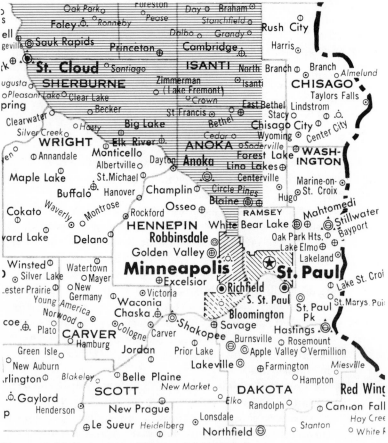

Figure 4 Market area of Memorial Hospital

Table 4 Market Share within Primary Service
Area of Memorial Hospital

Community*	% Market Share, by Total Days
Fridley	14.7
Spring Lake Park	18.3
Coon Rapids	46.8
Blaine	23.7
St. Francis-Bethel	37.2
Anoka	53.3
Champlin	48.3
Adjacent counties	
Isanti County	.8
Sherburne County	10.5
Wright County	.9

Source: PSRO data files on all patients in all
Minneapolis-St. Paul hospitals

*These communities represent 85% of Memorial
Hospital's admissions.

Issues

An important consideration in forecasting a hospital's future service area
is to acknowledge that it can have distinctly different geographic markets for each of its major inpatient and outpatient lines of business.
Graphically plotting each service's existing market area through an analysis of patient origin studies of either discharge or billing data files, as
well as records from the emergency department and outpatient clinics,
is imperative. Whether or not explicit market areas for every line of business are developed or whether an aggregate service area can be utilized for total admissions will depend on the availability of comparable
statistics from other providers. An important factor to determine is the
degree of competition that exists for the hospital's various lines of business. The greater the competition, the more targeted the marketing
should be and, therefore, the more detailed the segmentation and analysis of markets by each service.

The nature of the hospital's competitors for each line of business
also plays a role. The more competitors for each service and the more
aggressive they become, the more sophisticated and targeted forecasting, planning, and marketing should be. Other factors are the availability from within the hospital of detailed statistical data on patient origin

for each line of business and the interest and ability of the hospital's managers to utilize this information for decision-making purposes.

Forecasting the boundaries of future marketing areas is a function of the strategic planning process. Planning will identify whether marketing activities need to be strengthened in adjacent or remote geographic areas in order to protect existing markets or whether the hospital should diversify into new areas of projected growth. For most hospitals, as they first implement market-based forecasting, it is sufficient to use their existing primary service area as the geographic zone for future forecasting activities. This approach can be modified in future strategic planning and marketing cycles when the management group becomes more familiar and comfortable with the concepts and information.

Data

Information necessary for defining and forecasting service or market areas is usually available in hospital data files. The principal source of information will be discharge abstract information in the medical record department or statistical information stored in billing data files. Many hospitals maintain patient origin data by each of their major lines of business. These data should be classified by community and/or zip code.

The medical record department can be instructed to establish and maintain such data files. At least once a year, a computer analysis of billing information should be made to develop a statistical profile. Otherwise, other sources, such as patient origin studies conducted by local health planning agencies and hospital associations, analyses of Hospital Administrative Services or Professional Administrative Services reporting mechanisms (conducted by CPHA, Ann Arbor, MI), and analyses of data maintained by professional review organizations should be pursued.

Stage 2. Forecasting Market Population Profiles

A hospital's primary consumers are the actual users of its various services, that is, its physicians and patients. Other customers are those persons who materially influence another's use of the hospital's services. Physicians can be segmented and analyzed by age, specialty, office location, board status, affiliation with other hospitals, group or solo practice, admissions, patient days, ALOS, revenues, and affiliation with a preferred provider organization or health maintenance organization. (See appendix C for a discussion of demand forecasting that focuses on the admitting profiles and trends of medical staff.)

Patients can be segmented by types of services they have used in the past; by age, sex, and socioeconomic characteristics; and by source of payment and the geographic areas in which they live or work. Additional customers can be classified by the amount of influence they exert on the primary consumers.

Other demographic characteristics can also be gleaned from past customers by defining their socioeconomic class. In certain market areas, such additional features of the demographic profile are important because they can materially influence assumptions regarding future demand for various lines of business.

Unless there are large concentrations of differing socioeconomic groups, ageand sex-adjusted statistics will most likely capture the majority of demand variability within a service area.

Process

To develop and evaluate a demographic profile of customers, an analysis of the historical customer profile should be conducted by defining the age, sex, and payment source of past patients for each service or line of business. Memorial Hospital performed an analysis of customers by specialty (see table 5). This internal case mix was contrasted with the case mix for all patients hospitalized in the metropolitan area of Minneapolis-St. Paul. The profile suggests that Memorial has smaller proportions of medical-surgical patients than the metropolitan area as a whole, but slightly more obstetrical-gynecological and mental health and chemical dependency patients as a result of its inpatient programs in these areas.

Memorial Hospital also performed an analysis by customer age (see table 6). Approximately 12 percent of Memorial's customers are older than 65, and approximately 30 percent of its customers are younger than 18. This reflects the predominantly younger suburban population base in which Memorial is located. Approximately 60 percent of Memorial's customers are women, and approximately 30 percent of its customers have their bills paid by Medicare or Medicaid.

This understanding of characteristics of past customers provides a backdrop for projecting the characteristics of future customers.

The demographic profile of residents in the service or market area can only be defined using existing demographic analysis reports. A summary of population information for Memorial Hospital's service area and its forecasted growth (see table 7) demonstrates that in 1984 there were approximately 293,000 people living in the geographic area that

Table 5 Customer Profile for Memorial Hospital, by Inpatient Line of Business

Specialty	Memorial Hospital, %	Metropolitan Area, %
Cardiology	3.9	8.6
Psychiatry	6.7	4.6
Chemical dependency	4.6	3.0
Ophthalmology	1.4	2.4
Otorhinolaryngology	2.2	2.9
Neurology	3.0	2.0
Orthopedics	6.7	11.2
Urology	4.2	3.6
Gynecology	4.2	3.4
Obstetrics	16.5	10.6
Pediatrics	12.7	6.4
General medical and surgical	19.8	32.2
Newborns	14.1	8.9
Total	100.0	100.0

Source: PSRO data files for all metropolitan Minneapolis-St. Paul hospitals

Table 6 Customer Profile for Memorial Hospital, by Age

Age Group	Customer, %
Newborn	14.1
0–18	15.1
19–39	39.5
40–64	19.0
65 +	12.3
Total	100.0

Source: Memorial Hospital medical records

represents 85 percent of Memorial's inpatient demand. This geographic market area is expected to grow 22 percent between 1984 and 1994. These aggregate population statistics represent the potential customers for Memorial's lines of business in the future. And, the forecasts provide essential information for subsequent calculation of future utilization rates and aggregate demand for the market area.

Table 7 Forecasted Increases in Population

Community	1984	1994	% Increase	Average Annual Increase, %
Fridley	32,500	34,500	6.2	0.62
Spring Lake Park	7,000	7,000	0	0
Coon Rapids	37,500	46,200	23.2	2.32
Blaine	37,000	45,800	23.8	2.38
St. Francis-Bethel	11,350	12,700	11.9	1.19
Anoka	43,500	51,200	17.7	1.77
Champlin	15,280	19,890	30.2	3.02
Subtotal	184,130	217,290	18.0	1.80
Adjacent counties				
Isanti County	21,700	29,000	33.6	3.36
Sherburne County	32,100	41,200	28.3	2.83
Wright County	55,200	71,100	28.8	2.88
Subtotal	109,000	141,300	29.6	2.96
Total	293,130	358,590	22.3	2.23

Source: Minnesota State Demographer's Office

The Memorial market area has a high proportion of young persons, and the principal geographic region of Memorial's market area is Anoka County. Therefore, the forecasted age profile for this county is that only 6.6 percent of the population will be older than 65 in the year 2000 (see table 8). Comparing the Anoka market to the U.S. population for 1980, the Anoka market has considerably fewer persons older than 45 than the national average (see table 9).

Table 8 Percent Variations in Anoka County Age Profile, 1970 to 2000

Age Group	1970	1980	1990	2000
0–14	39.6	26.3	24.9	22.6
15–44	45.2	54.9	51.4	48.2
45–64	12.0	15.0	18.6	22.6
65+	3.2	3.8	5.1	6.6
Total	100	100	100	100

Source: Minnesota State Demographer's Office

Table 9 Comparative Analysis of Age in Anoka Market and U.S. Population

Age Group	Anoka County Population, %	U.S. Population, %
0–14	26.3	22.5
15–44	54.9	46.5
45–64	15.0	19.7
65 +	3.8	11.3
Total	100	100

Sources: U.S. Bureau of the Census and Minnesota State Demographer's Office (actual 1980 data, not adjusted)

Issues

Defining the geographic market area is an important consideration in forecasting the underlying population base for future demand forecasts. The definition can either be done by zip code or census tract. Census-tract boundaries should be used when analyzing historical population demographic trends and forecasting future population by age and sex cohorts. Although census-tract boundaries are customarily used for defining population of a market area, they are not necessarily identical to the zip code boundaries for the market area.

Because an important part of demand forecasting is integrating a hospital's historical utilization with historical population profiles, it is necessary to match utilization statistics with population statistics. If utilization statistics are developed on a zip-code basis, they should therefore be matched with population data developed on a census-tract basis. Computer software packages have been developed recently to assist in this matching process (see appendix A).

Most hospitals accept population forecasts from government agencies without question, but demographers can make mistakes or can base their forecasts on inappropriate assumptions of fertility rates and migration. It is therefore becoming increasingly important for hospital managers to understand the basic assumptions upon which future forecasts of population are based. A 10 percent error in the forecast of the number of residents in a market area, by age and sex, can significantly affect the expected demand for a hospital's lines of business.

Techniques used in forecasting cohort survival, utility connections, birth rate, migration, residence trends, and income adjusting are often based on wide and variable assumptions. Relatively inexpensive assistance can be secured from faculty in social science departments of local universities to analyze the population forecasts and their underlying forecasting methodologies or to adjust assumptions per the hospital manager's judgment.

Forecasting the racial composition and socioeconomic profile of a market area can be extremely important if any particular socioeconomic or racial group is concentrated in a market area. Poor groups tend to use hospital services differently than affluent groups. In most hospital market areas, however, forecasting based on age and sex should be sufficiently accurate for planning and marketing decisions.

In times of economic difficulty, the migration of major employers in and out of a hospital's market area can significantly affect not only the number and types of persons who might use the hospital's services, but also their ability to pay for these services. Therefore, forecasting future demographic characteristics should give consideration to any significant shift in the number and types of major employers and third-party payers. An increase in the number of high-risk industries and their work force can increase demand for outpatient and emergency services. Similarly, seasonal fluctuations in a predominantly tourist area will affect these same lines of business. Routine operational budgeting activities should anticipate such fluctuations in demand.

Data

Procurement of population and demographic analyses of market areas is considerably easier than other data-gathering tasks associated with hospital demand forecasting. Several sources exist from which to secure forecasts in demographic profiles. These are state and local planning agencies, state demographers' offices, local and regional economic development commissions, school districts, city planning offices, state and regional socioeconomic research firms, local health planning agencies, and the U.S. Bureau of the Census.

It is always prudent to secure population forecasts from more than one source in order to compare the forecasts for any variations. As has already been indicated, it is also desirable to gain understanding of the underlying assumptions upon which these population forecasts have been developed and to challenge their validity by using outside consultants or demographic advisors.

Stage 3. Forecasting Use Rates by Service

Definitions

The term *use rate* refers to the rate at which lines of business are utilized by certain customer groups. Use rates are usually measured as the number of units of service consumed per thousand persons for a given customer group or market segment. For hospitals, these are frequently stated in admissions per thousand or visits per thousand for each service or specialty. These utilization rates are a critical building block in the overall hospital demand forecasting process.

Hospital demand forecasting has relied historically on an aggregate admission rate per thousand; for example, the national average is approximately 167 per thousand for all population groups and all services. However, it will become increasingly important to develop use rates that are more specific to population groups and lines of business. There are four basic levels of specificity that hospital forecasting should take into consideration:

- *Level one, aggregate use rate.* For example, the national average for all population groups and all services for acute community hospitals is approximately 167 admissions per thousand.
- *Level two, aggregate specialty use rate.* For example, for all ages of both sexes a hospital's market area may have a cardiology use rate of 50 admissions per thousand persons.
- *Level three, sex-specific use rate.* For example, for all specialties in a specific market area, men have 40 admissions for thousand persons, whereas women have 35 admissions per thousand. This rate would be an important factor in developing age-and sex-specific use rates.
- *Level four, age- and sex-specific use rates.* For example, a hospital may find that its oncology utilization rate for men aged 45 to 64 is 30 admissions per thousand persons in contrast to 20 for women in the same age cohort.

Process

There are two methods that can be used to forecast use rates by service: a five-step process based on rates and a discharge rate technique.

Five-Step Process

The five important steps in the first method of developing use rates are as follows:

Step 1. Define the level of detail to be used in the forecasting process. Beginning as simply as possible is important. Once the management team's capability to handle more specific information evolves and as more comprehensive and accurate data bases become available, the process can expand to more sophisticated and specific use rates. In most communities, the aggregate use rate, or the specialty-specific use rate for the aggregate service area should be utilized. For example, the national average of 167 admissions per thousand persons should be age adjusted to estimate aggregate demand for inpatient activities. If the national demographic profile is accepted as average or normal for an area and the need or morbidity of that population is approximately the same as national disease incidence experience, national use rates can be used for local forecasting purposes. However, each county should have a specific use rate based upon its unique age and sex distribution.

Memorial Hospital should not use national use rates because its demographic profile is very different than the national average. The age distribution in Memorial's principal market area is considerably younger than the national distribution (see table 9). Memorial should therefore anticipate use rates that are less than the national average of 167 admissions per thousand. (In subsequent sections, the use rate in Memorial's area is shown to be 131 total admissions per thousand persons.)

These data can be age adjusted as follows. Using the data on the U.S. population demographic profile (see table 10) and the U.S. admissions by age and sex profile (see table 11), use rates can be calculated for all age cohorts. After age breakdowns are calculated as percentages of the hospital's service area (for Anoka County, see table 9), the age-adjusted use rate can be determined.

Age Cohort	Admissions	÷	Population	=	Use Rate
0–14	3,688		49,917		73.9
15–44	15,749		103,419		152.3
45–64	8,607		43,896		196.1
65+	9,096		24,977		364.2
	37,140		222,209		167.1

The calculations for Anoka County are as follows:

Area Use Rate/1000	×	Proportion of Anoka Population	=	Local Age-Adjusted Weighted Use Rate
73.9		0.263		19.44
152.3		0.541		82.39
196.1		0.150		29.42
364.2		0.038		13.84
				145.09

The expected value by age adjusting is 145.1, when rounded. The actual use rate for Anoka is 146.2. In this example, therefore, age adjust-

Table 10 Profile of U.S.
Population, by Age and Sex

Age and Sex Group	Population (thousands)
Male	
0–14	25,504
15–44	51,541
45–64	21,069
65 +	10,108
Subtotal	108,222
Female	
0–14	24,413
15–44	51,878
45–64	22,827
65 +	14,819
Subtotal	113,937
Total	
0–14	49,917
15–44	103,419
45–64	43,896
65 +	24,927
Total	222,159

Source: U.S. Bureau of the Census
(actual 1980 data, not adjusted)

ing provides an accurate use rate when additional data are not available. When more detail is available or can be developed, age adjusting
should be used only to estimate future demand roughly; when use-rate
data are available on a specialty-by-specialty basis, age adjusting provides a good cross-check.

Suburban hospitals operating in an extremely competitive environment should become familiar with the use of age- and sex-specific utilization rates for all major services and eventually age and sex use rates
by specialty or DRG. This additional level of sophistication will be necessary to target strategic marketing activities to enhance market share
within specific lines of business. Planning future resource allocation decisions without an understanding of expected demand for specific lines
of business is difficult, as is monitoring the success of marketing pro-

Table 11 U.S. Admission Experience, by Age and Sex

Age and Sex Group	Population (thousands)
Male	
0–14	2,078
15–44	4,855
45–64	4,030
65 +	3,936
Subtotal	14,899
Female	
0–14	1,610
15–44	10,894
45–64	4,577
65 +	5,160
Subtotal	22,241
Total	
0–14	3,688
15–44	15,749
45–64	8,607
65 +	9,096
Total	37,140
Admissions per 1,000	167

Source: U.S. Department of Health and Human Services, Center for Health Statistics (actual 1980 data, not adjusted)

grams to improve market share or broaden market base, unless shifts in demand and use rate by specialty and geographic area can be monitored. A hospital's data system should accommodate these data needs.

Step 2. Gather historical utilization information on inpatient and outpatient lines of business for all providers in the area. Developing a comprehensive and accurate data base on the number and types of admissions for all patients in all hospitals in the area is important. The number and types of emergency department and outpatient and clinic visits should also be included. In most communities, this task will not be easy. Sources of such data are PROs, health planning agencies, Medicare cost reports, county vital statistics records, hospital annual reports, insurance data files, or market research studies asking where people went for which types of service and when.

Step 3. Match historical utilization statistics with corresponding population groups or years under consideration. Developing a use rate by dividing the total number of admissions for the market area in 1984 by the population that existed in 1980 would be totally inappropriate. It is critical that the population data appearing in the denominator of the use rate be developed for the same types of people and year as the utilization data that appears in the numerator. For example, the use rate for an obstetrical line of business should not be calculated by dividing the number of obstetrical admissions by the entire population, both male and female, but rather by the number of women in the childbearing years of 15 to 44.

Step 4. Prepare and publish utilization rates by the smallest geographic or demographic unit feasible. Calculating an aggregate utilization rate for Memorial Hospital's market area demonstrates that, for the 1984 population of approximately 293,000, approximately 38,000 admissions were generated, that is, an aggregate utilization rate of 131 admissions per thousand persons (see table 12). This utilization rate is considerably lower than the national average of 167 admissions per thousand and could be the result of Memorial's relatively young demographic characteristics. This discrepancy also may be a function of the relatively healthy nature of this rapidly growing suburban market area and the role that health maintenance organizations are beginning to play in the market area.

Memorial Hospital also employs a strategy for estimating utilization rates for all patients of all geographic regions when actual data are not available (see table 12). The admission profile was derived by conducting a one-month sample for all hospitals in the market area. This one-month sample was annualized and, therefore, the potential exists for error to have been incorporated in these forecasts. Inasmuch as hospital demand forecasting is in its infancy in the United States, hospital managers should acknowledge this potential error and establish cooperative arrangements with neighboring hospitals to improve the availability of and access to more comprehensive and accurate data bases in the future.

Memorial attempted to extrapolate the utilization rate of the suburban portion of its market area from the portions of rural counties neighboring the metropolitan area. The assignment of a use rate of 131 admissions per thousand to these suburban fringe communities may also include some error, although it is based on *similar* age and sex distributions. If the age distributions had been significantly different, this

Table 12 Estimated Use Rates for All Diagnoses, 1984

Community	Population	Admissions	Estimated Use Rate
Fridley	32,500	3,793	116.7
Spring Lake Park	7,000	740	105.7
Coon Rapids	37,500	4,294	114.5
Blaine	37,000	4,429	119.7
St. Francis-Bethel	11,350	1,825	160.8
Anoka	43,500	6,360	146.2
Champlin	15,280	2,695	176.4
Subtotal	184,130	24,136	131.1*
Adjacent counties			
Isanti County	21,700	2,849	131.3
Sherburne County	32,100	4,215	131.3
Wright County	55,200	7,248	131.3
Subtotal	109,000	14,312	131.3
Total	293,130	38,448	131.2

Source: PSRO data files for Minneapolis-St. Paul hospitals and a statewide patient origin study, conducted by the Minnesota Hospital Association, of a one-month sample of discharges for all hospitals

*The average use rate in the subtotal row will be used for all areas outside the metropolitan area, based upon similar age distributions.

methodology would have been unacceptable. These potential weaknesses in the accuracy in demand forecasts for Memorial must be taken into consideration. Forecasting is not designed to eliminate error, but it is important that a hospital's forecasting process at least make explicit all assumptions utilized in the development of statistical indexes and acknowledge, wherever appropriate, those areas that may be the most susceptible to error.

Age- and sex-specific utilization rates for the United States can be used within an individual hospital service area only with extreme caution. Because utilization rates by age and sex cohort vary dramatically among regions of the United States, national data that are broken down regionally often prove more accurate than aggregate U.S. data and should be used when available. It is also imperative to recall that utilization rates vary significantly by specialty. A particular hospital's market area may experience dramatically different use rates than might be evident in these national statistics or in the Memorial Hospital market area. However, when regional data are not available, an estimate of the number of general acute care admissions to community hospitals in the United States by age and sex cohort can be used. Dividing these admission profiles (obtained from table 11) by the population for each of these age and sex cohorts (obtained from table 10) obtains the age and sex use rates (see table 13).

Step 5. Prepare and publish utilization rates by specialty for the hospital's market area. Memorial Hospital is interested in developing specialty-specific use rates for its market area. These data are not readily available because detailed information on a diagnosis or specialty-specific basis has not been published in a format that facilitates the development of specialty-specific use rates. The managers of Memorial have elected to develop estimates of these use rates by calculating the number of admissions in the market area by specialty first and then dividing these expected admissions by known population information in order to get use rates measured in admissions per thousand.

Table 13 U.S. Age and Sex Use Rates per 1,000[a]

Age and Sex Group	Admissions (thousands)	Population (thousands)	Use Rate[b] per 1,000
Male			
0–14	2,078	25,504	81.5
15–44	4,855	51,541	94.2
45–64	4,030	21,069	191.3
65+	3,936	10,108	389.4
Subtotal	14,899	108,222	137.7
Female			
0–14	1,610	24,413	65.9
15–44	10,894	51,878	210.0
45–64	4,577	22,827	200.5
65+	5,160	14,819	348.2
Subtotal	22,241	113,937	195.2
Total			
0–14	3,688	49,917	73.9
15–44	15,749	103,419	152.3
45–64	8,607	43,896	196.1
65+	9,096	24,927	364.9
Total	37,140	222,159	167.2

[a]Actual 1980 data, not adjusted.
[b]Use rate = admissions experience ÷ population × 1,000.

Memorial estimated the specialty admissions for its aggregate market area for all patients and all hospitals as follows. Memorial knew that its market area generated approximately 38,000 total admissions in 1984 (see table 12). Assuming that the specialty distribution of these admissions is similar to the specialty distribution for the aggregate metropolitan area, the proportion of admissions in oncology, cardiology, and other specialties can be estimated. The metropolitan case mix of patients multiplied by 38,447 admissions yields the aggregate service area admission profile for that specialty (see table 14). For example, given the fact that 5.7 percent of the metropolitan area's admissions were in oncology services, this suggests that 2,200 oncology admissions would be demanded in Memorial's service area. Obviously, this estimate is valid only if the actual morbidity or demand pattern of Memorial's market area (the northwestern quadrant of the metropolitan area) is sufficiently similar to the overall metropolitan case-mix profile. This is another instance where error may be injected into the forecasting process and, accordingly, the underlying assumptions associated with this calculation must be made explicit to Memorial's managers and other parties using the forecasts.

Table 14 Specialty Admissions for Memorial Market Area, 1984

Specialty	Metropolitan Distribution, %[a]	Estimate of Aggregate Admissions
Oncology	5.7	2,200
Cardiology	8.6	3,330
Psychiatry	4.6	1,770
Chemical dependency	3.0	1,155
Ophthalmology	2.4	925
Enterology	2.9	1,115
Neurology	2.0	780
Orthopedics	11.2	4,310
Urology	3.6	1,390
Gynecology	3.4	1,310
Obstetrics	10.6	4,075
Pediatrics	6.4	2,465
General medical and surgical	26.5	10,200
Newborns	8.9	3,422
Total	100.0[b]	38,447

[a]PSRO data for all patients in all Minneapolis-St. Paul hospitals, January through June 1984.

[b]Actual value is 99.8%; the discrepancy is the result of rounding.

Given the distribution of admissions by specialty the utilization rates for Memorial's market area can be calculated (see table 15). Dividing 3,330 cardiology admissions by the aggregate population in the Memorial market area of 293,130 yields a cardiology use rate in this market area of 11.361 admissions per thousand persons.

The specialty-specific use rate is important in the forecasting of future demand for cardiology business in the Memorial market area because, as the total population within Memorial's market area increases in the future, the number of cardiology admissions (all things being equal) would be expected to rise at the rate of 11 admissions for every increase per thousand persons older than 15 in the market area.

The use rates for obstetrics and gynecology were developed by dividing estimated obstetrics admissions by the number of women in the population, not aggregate population. Similarly, the pediatric use rate of 31.97 was derived by dividing estimated admissions of children under

Table 15 Use Rates in Memorial Market Area, by Specialty, 1984

Specialty	Total Area Admissions[a]	Aggregate Population	Estimated Use Rate (thousands)[b]
Cardiology	3,330		11.36
Medicine, oncology, surgery, and dental surgery	12,400		42.30
Obstetrics	4,075		27.26[c]
Gynecology	1,310		8.76[c]
Urology	1,390		4.74
Orthopedics	4,310		14.70
Neurology	780		2.66
Otorhinolaryngology	1,115		3.80
Ophthalmology	925		3.16
Mental health	1,770		6.034
Chemical dependency	1,155		3.94
Pediatrics (under 14)	2,465		31.97[c]
Newborns	3,422		11.67
Total	38,447	293,130	131.2

[a]From table 14.
[b]Assumes even distribution of age and sex cohorts throughout the area and specialties.
[c]Determined by dividing admissions by the total number of women or children, as appropriate, in the target market area.

14 years by the total number of children under 14 years in the market area.

Development and use of use rates will not always comply with the degree of specificity and sophistication that managers might wish. For example, a curious amalgam of admissions associated with general medicine, oncology, general surgery, and dental surgery results in a relatively large use rate (see table 15). A rate such as this is less desirable than a use rate that could be made specific for general medicine and a use rate specific to oncology, general surgery, and dental surgery. Nevertheless, it is important to begin developing and using use rates at whatever level of detail is available. As managers expand their interest and ability to use more specific data and as more comprehensive and accurate data bases become available, more sophisticated forecasting activities will be possible.

Discharge Rate Technique

Many hospitals have found that the challenge of securing accurate statistical information on admissions or discharges from other hospitals in their market area has stimulated them to develop demand forecasting models based on their own data files. This technique has been used for several years by hospital planners and consulting organizations and is referred to here as the *discharge rate technique* because it is the ratio of a hospital's discharges to the unique population base in its market area. Therefore, the discharge rate equals the number of admissions divided by the population in the market area.

For example, if 50 percent of Memorial Hospital's 10,000 admissions (that is, 5,000 admissions) came from the community that had 100,000 persons residing in it, the discharge rate for this particular community would be 50 admissions per thousand population. Specialty-specific or service-specific discharge ratios can be similarly calculated and used to forecast future demand by multiplying these discharge rates times anticipated future population forecasts. Although this technique can be used as a proxy indicator of future demand, it has a number of methodological flaws that must be acknowledged and guarded against. The discharge ratio must be modified to take into consideration anticipated changes in underlying shifts that might be occurring in various age and sex cohorts. And, most important, assumptions about market share should be revised. If a hospital's use rate is held constant from 1980 to 1990 and the population increases for a specific geographic area during this same period, the hospital would anticipate a substantial increase in number of admissions. However, achieving the expected admissions will happen only if the market share remains at least what it was in 1980.

Issues

Several important considerations must be explicitly addressed in the development and use of improved use-rate forecasting methodologies:

Level of detail. Utilization rates must be manageable during development and understandable and usable once they are generated. Statistical indexes or data that are not easily adapted to decision-making activities are wasted.

Appropriate matching. It is imperative that historical utilization statistics be matched with the appropriate population group. This match must be for the appropriate year, as well. There should also be some logical linkage between the utilization data and the underlying characteristics of the population group. For example, an obstetrical use rate for all women or for women of childbearing age is preferable to an obstetrical use rate for total population.

Intercensal population estimates. Hospitals will frequently find that they have utilization statistics for a year that may not have readily available population information. This difficulty can be overcome in two ways: Straight-line extrapolation of population data can be developed for intercensal years, or, the hospital can pay particular attention to the development of historical utilization in those years for which solid population information is more readily available, that is, 1970, 1975, and 1980.

Trends and use rates. It is not desirable to develop a single use rate for a single year. Use rates change at varying rates over time and by specialty. As the population ages, use rates for chronic diseases have been increasing. The exact rate of change varies in the United States and, therefore, evaluating use rates for the prior three years within a market area is imperative. This evaluation of historical trends and use rates can be considered a starting point for extrapolating assumptions about how these use rates might change in the future.

Data on all patients from all hospitals. Securing valid data on all patients from all hospitals in a service area is difficult. A number of data sources exist at the national, regional, and state levels. They can be used to secure utilization rates suitable for the development of at least aggregate use rates per thousand population. Development of service or specialty-specific use rates by age and sex is considerably more difficult. Close cooperation among neighboring hospitals is important. If a full year of statistics cannot be secured easily, cooperation among hospitals to conduct one-month or two-month sample analyses of discharge abstracts would be desirable.

In-and-out migration. A source of potential error in the development of use rates for a market area can occur when there are substantial admissions of people residing outside this market area. Hospitals that rely on a wide variety of subspecialty lines of business usually draw patients from large geographic markets. The extent to which a hospital relies on admissions from distant communities will dictate the amount of difficulty it will have in calculating reliable use rates for its principal market area versus use rates from secondary referral areas. This variation should be taken into consideration when developing use rates and applying them to the market area population. In the case of Memorial Hospital, approximately 15 percent of inpatients reside outside of its principal market area. Use rates developed for its principal market area can be applied to the population base of its market area. Estimates of future demand from the distant areas should be calculated.

Data

Although it is not easy to secure actual utilization data in the quantity and format most desirable, there are several sources of information that will prove helpful. Possible sources of data are as follows:

- An analysis of discharge abstracts can be conducted for all patient admissions in all hospitals in the market area for comparable periods during the past three years. Such a study could be sponsored by the state or local hospital association or directly with neighboring hospitals.
- The *American Hospital Association Guide to the Health Care Field*, published annually by the American Hospital Association, Chicago, can be used to secure aggregate patient days for the market area, which then can be converted to admissions.
- Statistical information can be purchased from local PROs and analyzed by computer. If only federal data are available, the use rates developed will relate to the Medicare or Medicaid population groups. Although it is difficult to extrapolate use patterns of these population groups to all other age and sex cohorts, improved accuracy in forecasting demand from these markets (generally 30 percent to 50 percent of business) would put a hospital in a stronger operating position than had no forecast of future demand been done for any population group.
- Analyses can be made of third-party payer billing files from either Blue Cross or other commercial insurance carriers. Confidentiality of individual physicians, patients, and hospitals might preclude gaining access to the level of detail desired. However, aggregate admitting or discharge statistics for the area would facilitate developing areawide use rates. The development of areawide admission profiles for given periods also enables calculation of market share of the aggregate admitting profiles by dividing

admissions from a defined area by the expected total admissions
from that same area and that same period.

- The American Hospital Association, state hospital associations,
and various research organizations are increasingly utilizing statistics made available from national surveys conducted by the U.S.
Department of Health and Human Services, Center for Health
Statistics.
- An increasingly sophisticated data base is being developed by
many of the discharge abstracting services in the United States.
Statistical analyses that could be adapted for the hospital's market area can be purchased from these organizations.

Stage 4: Forecasting Aggregate Customer Demand for Each Service

Definitions

Aggregate customer demand is the total number of admissions or visits that
are estimated to occur in a specific area during a specific time in the
future. These expected utilization patterns can be forecasted for either
an entire service or market area or for individual components of the geographic market. In 1980, Memorial Hospital had 38,000 admissions from
a specific geographic market. This represents the aggregate market or
total demand for all lines of hospital inpatient business. The important
issue for a hospital's management team, however, is what proportion
of this aggregate market will decide actually to use the hospital's services. This question of market share is addressed during stage 5 of the
overall demand forecasting process.

The aggregate customer demand in a hospital's primary market area
may be stated in as much detail as managers are comfortable using and
for which data and information are readily available. However, in the
future, hospitals will need to forecast aggregate customer demand not
just for generic or average hospital inpatient and outpatient services,
but also for each line of business. For example, it will become necessary to forecast the total number of cardiology admissions expected for
the market area for future years, and then ultimately to determine what
proportion of that aggregate will be served by the hospital.

In the case of Memorial Hospital, the forecasted population expected
to reside in the market area by 1994 is approximately 358,000. The various geographic areas within this region have forecasted population
figures that can be applied against the expected use rate for 1994. If during the development of the base-case forecast for Memorial Hospital the
assumption is made that the 1994 use rate will be identical to the 1980

use rate, the estimated aggregate number of admissions for the market area in 1994 can be calculated (see table 16). With an average use rate of 131.3 per thousand population, the 358,590 persons expected to reside in the market area in 1994 will generate approximately 47,000 admissions. Thus, a 22 percent increase in admissions is expected to occur in the market area from 1984 to 1994 (see table 17). This is identical to the population increase, which demonstrates that when the use rate is held constant, the only determinant of future demand is the relative increase or decrease in population. Specialty-specific age and sex use rates, however, are desirable because they facilitate consideration of changes that could be occurring in the underlying demographic profile of the market area or the morbidity patterns of a population base.

Forecasting aggregate demand for a hospital's market area should also take into consideration the implications of potential fluctuations that result from migration of persons living and working in the market area. Depending on the unique nature of the demographic profile of the area and the economic environment associated with jobs, housing, transportation, and other factors, there could be as high as a 5 percent fluctua-

Table 16 Estimated Admissions for Memorial Hospital Market Area, 1994

Community	Population	Use Rate	Estimated Admissions*
Fridley	34,500	116.7	4,026
Spring Lake Park	7,000	105.7	740
Coon Rapids	46,200	114.5	5,290
Blaine	45,800	119.7	5,482
St. Francis-Bethel	12,700	160.8	2,042
Anoka	51,200	146.2	7,485
Champlin	19,890	176.4	3,509
Subtotal	217,290	131.3	28,574
Adjacent counties			
Isanti County	29,000	131.3	3,808
Sherburne County	41,200	131.3	5,410
Wright County	71,100	131.3	9,335
Subtotal	141,300	131.3	18,553
Total	385,590	131.3	47,127

*Population X estimated use rate = estimated admissions for the service area.

Table 17 Expected Growth in Admissions for Total Market Area, 1984 to 1994

	1984	1994	Change, %
Total market area admissions	38,447	47,127	22.58*
Population	293,130	358,590	22.33*
Use rate per 1,000	131.3	131.3	0

*Rounding precludes identical growth rates.

tion in future population. Aggregate demand for the area can also fluctuate if hospitals within the market have large subspecialty tertiary care referral patterns developed outside of the geographic service area, or referral patterns developed outside of the geographic boundaries of the defined primary market area.

The base-case forecast of hospital demand must, therefore, assume that previous in-and-out migration patterns will remain constant. Any assumed variations should be explicitly defined and explained.

Age- and sex-specific use rates or specialty use rates would be multiplied by corresponding population forecasts for the appropriate age and sex cohort. This calculation is straightforward and does not require sophisticated computer processing, unless there are a large number of specific use rates for a particular line of business, many age and sex cohorts, or many components of the defined market area.

Issues

Determination of future aggregate demand for a hospital's market area can be frustrated by a lack of statistical data from neighboring hospitals also serving the same area. As previously discussed, the alternate discharge rate can be used to extrapolate future demand for the service and then to calculate the hospital's expected share of that market. The most effective forecasting model calculates aggregate demand for the overall market first and then calculates the hospital's relative share of that market. This is the best model for two important reasons: (1) Future hospital operating environments will be characterized by intense competition among many providers for each line of business, and, (2) In an increasingly competitive environment, hospital managers will be developing and using decision-making processes for strategic planning and marketing that will target key marketing strategies for priority market groups and market areas.

Forecasting models must facilitate managers' capacity to pose "what if" questions throughout these planning and marketing processes. The forecasting process must also provide sufficient sensitivity so that decision making can be directed at several decision points and at the several variables that influence a market's and a hospital's demand. The forecasting model defined within this book is, therefore, a "market-based" approach guided by these principles.

Data

Data required to accomplish the calculations in stage 4 are obtained from the outputs of stage 2 and stage 3. Data made available during these previous stages are integrated in stage 4 to calculate future hospital demand for either inpatient or outpatient lines of business. The calculation of demand for emergency department and various outpatient clinic services parallels the process described for inpatient services.

Stage 5: Forecasting Market Share for Each Customer Group

Definitions

A hospital's market share represents that proportion of the aggregate demand in a defined market that has been or for which it is reasonable to assume will be served by the hospital. It is generally measured in terms of the number of admissions or visits that the hospital actually will receive from the market area versus those customers who may choose to use other providers serving the same market. Market share usually is presented as a percentage by major service or specialty.

Most hospitals are not comfortable with considering their services as lines of business that compete for distinctly different markets and that require very different marketing strategies. It will be imperative for hospital managers in the future to become more familiar with planning and monitoring their utilization performance by monitoring subtle changes in market share within defined geographic areas for each discrete line of business and to better understand the interrelationships between those services or lines of business.

Market share varies considerably by service, type of customer, and geographic distance from the hospital. A hospital's market share is a function of distance from the facility (see figure 5). In communities where geographic markets are remote from a hospital, those hospitals will have considerably less market share than in those communities that are closer to the hospital. Another important variable is the hospital's proximity to prime competitors. It is not uncommon for a referral hospital with little competition to draw patients from 100 or more miles. Patients can also migrate within highly competitive areas.

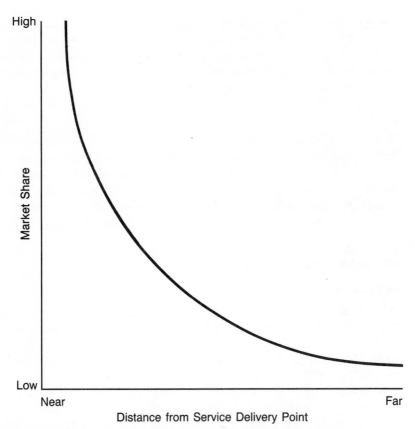

Figure 5 Market share relationship to proximity to hospital

Taking this relationship between market share and proximity to the service delivery point into consideration is appropriate for all lines of business. Subspecialty or tertiary care facilities rely on a broader geographic area to secure 85 percent of admissions volume. However, the relative market share at the periphery would still be similar to the market share proportions of other hospitals for other types of services. An important point in tracking consumers is that they will be more likely to travel for tertiary care than for obstetrical care and other services for which decisions are often based upon convenience. Therefore, forecasting market share must take into consideration such factors as the distance from the delivery point of various populations and the features of the services themselves.

The ability to achieve high proportions of any given market obviously will be influenced by the number and competitiveness of other hospital and health care providers attempting to serve the same market area. Expected market share objectives will vary by the type of facility, service, and certainly nature of the competitive environment within which a given hospital is operating (see figure 6). In certain subspecialty services, a teaching center would anticipate receiving a much higher share of tertiary markets than might other community hospitals unable to provide intricate subspecialty technology and staffing requirements. Rural hospitals that have a balance of primary care practitioners and

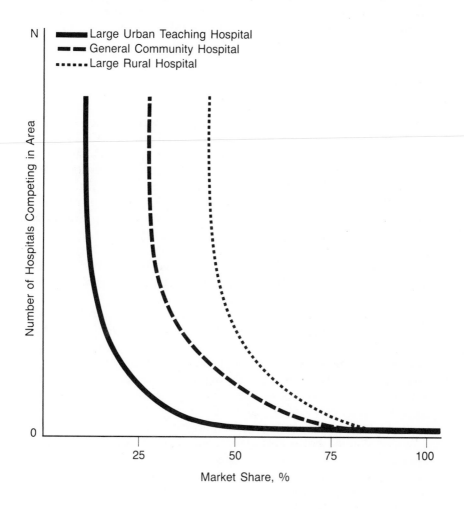

Figure 6 Variability of expected market share objectives

specialists on their medical staff would find it easier to achieve higher market share objectives by virtue of their stronger position in a less competitive environment.

Process

In probing the experience of Memorial Hospital, not just shifts in market share for total admissions should be monitored, but also fluctuations in market share for specific lines of business. In forecasting market share for each line of business, there are two basic strategies to be considered: calculation of *actual* market share statistics and the development of "synthetic" market share.

Actual Market Share

The process for developing actual market share indexes requires that, for a given line of business and a given geographic market, data are available on all admissions for all patients from all providers for a defined period. If a specific census tract or market area generated 100 admissions with one hospital accommodating 20 of those admissions, that hospital obviously received a 20 percent share of that particular market. Although most hospitals have been struggling to determine their market share for the total number of general admissions, market share for each specialty also should be calculated. Market share indicators for each line of business must also be tracked longitudinally. The development of market share trends for at least three years will be an essential backdrop of information for anticipating expected trends in future market share performance.

Data for a three-month period in 1984 suggest that, for the principle communities within the primary market area of Memorial Hospital, 35,290 admissions were generated (see table 18). Of these aggregate number of admissions, Memorial Hospital responded to the needs of 5,250 persons, or 14.9 percent, of the aggregate market. Memorial's market share varies considerably among its several communities. During the period from 1978 to 1984, Memorial lost market share in five of seven communities and made modest gains in two communities (see table 19). Available data do not enable determining whether this is a real shift in market share or a function of different statistical techniques applied to different data bases, and, therefore, this relative slip in market share must be explored further.

Table 18 Memorial Hospital Market Share, April through June 1984

Community	Total Patients, All Hospitals, All Diagnoses	All Diagnoses	Memorial Market Share, %
Columbia Heights	1,579	63	4.0
Fridley	2,086	177	8.5
Spring Lake Park	407	39	9.6
Coon Rapids	2,361	1,240	52.5
Blaine	2,436	565	23.2
St. Francis-Bethel	1,004	405	40.3
Anoka	3,497	1,789	51.2
Columbus	184	61	33.2
Camden	2,704	39	1.4
N.E. Minneapolis	3,688	41	1.1
Near North	2,363	52	2.2
Brooklyn Center	4,533	14	0.3
Brooklyn Park	3,031	74	0.2
Champlin	1,483	507	34.2
West Hennepin	1,441	56	3.9
New Brighton	1,588	69	4.3
Mounds View	905	59	6.5
Total	35,290	5,250	14.9

Source: PSRO data base for all patients in Minneapolis-St. Paul metropolitan hospitals

Table 19 Trends in Market Share of Memorial Hospital

Community	Market Share 1978[a]	Market Share 1984[b]	Direction of Change
Fridley	14.7	8.5	Down
Spring Lake Park	18.3	9.6	Down
Coon Rapids	46.8	52.5	Up
Blaine	23.7	23.2	Down
St. Francis-Bethel	37.2	40.3	Up
Anoka	53.3	51.2	Down
Champlin	48.3	34.2	Down

[a]From HSA patient origin study for November 1978.

[b]From table 18.

Synthetic Market Share

With regard to obstetrical activities, hospitals can calculate the market share by going to county vital statistics records to determine the number of births at specific hospitals during defined periods. A specific hospital will then find it a fairly straightforward process to determine the proportion of these births on record that occurred within its facility. Synthetic extrapolation techniques will be necessary for other services. Information on aggregate admissions can be secured from the *AHA Guide to the Health Care Field*, published by the American Hospital Association, Chicago, and by procuring and analyzing hospital Medicare cost reports for a defined market area.

In addition, market research techniques can be employed in which random-sample surveys are conducted to identify which hospitals residents of the area have used and for what services (see appendix B for a sample research instrument). These types of statistical analyses can be valuable in generalizing market share information, given statistically valid research design and sampling techniques.

Issues

Two recurring issues in the demand forecasting model are evident in the market share arena: (1) the availability of comprehensive and accurate data on all patients and providers in a defined area for a defined period, and (2) attention to the level of detail actually required and used by management for strategic planning and marketing purposes. The more sophisticated the detail of the data must be to satisfy managers, the more difficult it will be to assemble and maintain statistical information suitable for the forecasting functions. Synthetic market share information will be developed in many communities by extrapolating from reports published by local hospitals or area planning bodies.

Data

Statistical information potentially necessary for forecasting market share indicators includes original research into physicians' views of the proportion of the market that will come to the hospital for defined lines of business (this can be done in structured interviews, but would have the added difficulty of potential error and bias). Conducting structured interviews or market research surveys of the general population to determine historical and future market share estimates is also potentially necessary.

These market research inquiries also have the added advantage of gathering additional subjective information in an attempt to explain why market share indicators are at the level suggested by the respondents, and to identify additional strategies to broaden market base or expand market share.

Information is also available from the *AHA Guide*, Medicare cost reports, PRO data tapes, tapes from third-party payers, cooperative patient origin studies conducted by neighboring hospitals, county vital statistics offices, and various local and state health planning bodies.

Stage 6: Forecasting a Future Utilization Profile

Definitions

The utilization profile represents the forecasted demand for each of the hospital's major lines of business. This demand is frequently measured in terms of the number of admissions or visits and is the ultimate forecast of the number and type of patients the hospital will serve at any given time in the near future.

Process

The methodology used to forecast demand for specific hospital services is not complicated and relies on straightforward logic. Market share indicators identified in stage 5 are multiplied by aggregate demand dealt with in stage 4. Breaking down aggregate demand and market share by lines of business yields the anticipated demand for each of those services.

Memorial Hospital's experience illustrates the calculations associated with stage 6 (see table 20). In 1984, the primary market area for Memorial Hospital generated 38,446 admissions. However, Memorial received only 11,087 of these, or a market share of approximately 29 percent. In addition to the admissions from its primary market area, Memorial received an additional 2,400 admissions from market areas outside the principle service area, for a total demand of 13,487 admissions for its various inpatient lines of business.

Assuming that the 1984 market share holds constant to the year 1994, the demand in 1994 will be 13,561 admissions from the primary market area and an additional 2,777 from the others, for a total demand for future inpatient lines of business of 16,338 admissions. Using these assumptions on market share, Memorial can expect a 21 percent increase in its inpatient business between 1984 and 1994. Similar calculations can be employed on a market share basis for each line of business, if data are available. These calculations will result in the expected number of admissions for each inpatient service in 1994.

Table 20 Demand after Considering Market Share
of Memorial Hospital

Community	Aggregate Admissions		% Market Share, 1984*	Memorial Demand		% Change
	1984	1994		1984	1994	
Fridley	3,793	4,026	8.5	322	342	
Spring Lake Park	740	740	9.6	71	71	
Coon Rapids	4,293	5,290	52.5	2,254	2,777	
Blaine	4,429	5,482	23.2	1,028	1,272	
St. Francis-Bethel	1,825	2,042	40.3	735	823	
Anoka	6,358	7,485	51.2	3,255	3,832	
Champlin	2,696	3,509	34.2	922	1,200	
Subtotal	24,134	28,574	35.6	8,587	10,317	20
Adjacent counties						
Isanti County	2,849	3,808	20	570	762	
Sherburne County	4,215	5,410	20	843	1,082	
Wright County	7,248	9,335	15	1,087	1,400	
Subtotal	14,312	18,553	17.5	2,500	3,244	30
Subtotal	38,446	47,127	28.8	11,087	13,561	22
Other areas	—	—	—	2,400	2,777	16
Total	38,446	47,127	N/A	13,487	16,338	21

*From table 18.

Memorial Hospital developed forecasts for specialty admissions in 1994 by assuming that the hospital case-mix distribution would remain virtually the same during a 10-year period. This assumption could be dangerous if during these 10 years, Memorial adds any new services or physicians. Fluctuations in the activities of individual physicians and in the proportion of medical staff assigned to various specialty areas can dramatically influence case mix from one year to the next. Acknowledging these potential sources of error can help hospital managers guard against inappropriate interpretations in their future demand forecast profiles.

Many hospitals will find it difficult to gain access to market share information because of the lack of cooperation and lack of data from other providers. However, because dramatic differences in gross and net revenues make it desirable to anticipate future demand by specialty or service, synthetic methods are necessary to generate anticipated case-mix forecasts for the inpatient lines of business.

Extrapolating from historical data to forecast future demand by specialty group is an example of how a hospital can implement synthetic methods (see table 21). The assumption that market share use rate or case mix will not change during 10 years is probably unreasonable. Ultimately, this assumption and the forecast should be modified in response to additional studies made during the strategic planning and marketing process (see chapter 4 on future scenario development and its impact on future demand).

Table 21 Demand at Memorial Hospital, by Specialty, 1984 to 1994

Specialty Diagnosis	Case Mix, FY 1984, %	Admissions, 1984	Forecasted Admissions, 1994
Adults (older than 18)			
Cardiology	3.9	526	637
Medicine	10.7	1,444	1,748
Surgery	9.1	1,228	1,487
Obstetrics	16.5	2,225	2,696
Gynecology	4.2	592	686
Urology	4.2	566	686
Orthopedics	6.7	904	1,095
Neurology	3.0	405	490
Dental surgery	0.2	27	33
Otorhinolaryngology	2.2	297	359
Ophthalmology	1.4	189	229
Mental health	5.4	728	882
Chemical dependency	4.5	607	735
Subtotal	72.0	9,738	11,763
Pediatrics (up to 18)			
Psychology	1.3	175	212
Chemical dependency	0.1	13	16
Gynecology	0.2	26	32
Other diagnosis	12.3	1,659	2,010
Subtotal	13.9	1,873	2,270
Newborn	14.1	1,902	2,304
Total	100.0	13,513	16,337

Sources: Memorial Hospital medical records and table 18

The purpose of these preliminary base-case forecasts, however, is to test future consequences of plans and strategies already in place in Memorial Hospital. If these plans and management actions do not change and if Memorial's position in its competitive marketplace does not change, the driving force for increases or decreases in future demand will be driven principally by fluctuations in the population base. Forecasting calculations should reflect such fluctuations.

Issues

Forecasting future demand for hospitals is complicated and dependent on several assumptions made about key variables. As the forecasting model proceeds with calculations related to population, historical utilization, use rates, and market share, the potential for error increases.

Several important junctures in the forecasting process must be explicitly identified and considered by all planning and marketing participants. Identification of these various assumptions at an explicit level will facilitate healthy debate and discussion about the nature of future demand among the planning and marketing participants. It also enables the participants to reach a consensus about action to take to influence the variables important in driving future demand for a hospital's lines of business.

Data

The results of stages 4 and 5 are necessary to perform the steps in stage 6. Market share forecasts are multiplied by aggregate demand forecasts to determine forecasts of expected utilization for inpatient and outpatient lines of business.

To assist Memorial's strategic planning and marketing activities, future demand forecasts should be made not only for 1980 and 1990, but also for critical years in between. Detailed population data generally are available on a year-by-year basis. If specific assumptions can be made about use rate and market share for each year, the forecasting methodology outlined above can be applied to forecast future demand for various lines of business for each year between 1980 and 1990.

Demand in the interval years can be estimated by developing a straight-line interpolation between the demand forecasts for 1994 and the base year of 1984. Modifications to this straight-line assumption obviously can be made if there are indications in the hospital's market area that the rate of growth might be greater or less than the anticipated straight-line growth. Assumptions about the rate of change of this demand should be explicit and challenged by all participants in the strategic planning and marketing processes. For example, the demand pro-

Table 22 Extrapolated Demand at Memorial Hospital, by Specialty, 1984 to 1994[a]

Specialty	Admissions										
	1984	1985	1986	1987	1988	1989	1990	1991	1992	1993	1994
Cardiology	526					582					637
Medicine	1,444					1,596					1,748
Surgery	1,228					1,358					1,487
Obstetrics	2,225					2,461					2,696
Gynecology	592					655					718
Urology	566					626					686
Orthopedics	904					1,000					1,096
Neurology	405					448					490
Dental surgery	27					30					33
Otorhinolaryngology	297					328					359
Ophthalmology	189					209					229
Mental health	903					998					1,094
Chemical dependency	620					685					751
Pediatrics	1,659					1,848					2,010
Newborn	1,902					2,103					2,304
Total	13,487					14,927[b]					16,338

[a]From table 21; assumes straight-line growth from 1984 to 1994 and no change in use rate, market share, or case mix.

[b]A 10.67% increase over 1984.

file for Memorial Hospital in 1989 is 14,927 admissions distributed among several specialty lines of business (see table 22). The 1989 demand profile represents a 10.67 percent increase over the demand profile for 1984. (This 1989 demand forecast will serve as the focal point for subsequent application in the forecasting methods of stages 7 through 9.)

Stage 7: Forecasting Average Length of Stay for Each Inpatient Service

Definitions

Average length of stay (ALOS) represents the average number of days that the average patient remains in a hospital. Average lengths of stay differ among the various types of admissions.

In general, the ALOS for most specialties has been declining throughout the United States. Even for the one-year period from 1983 to 1984, Memorial Hospital experienced a drop in ALOS from 7.51 days to 6.94 days (see table 23). This drop was similar to the trend for all hospitals within the metropolitan area, which was 7.81 days in 1983 and 7.75 days in 1984.

Memorial Hospital has a dramatic variation in ALOS for various specialties (see table 24). These range from a high of 17 days per admission for a mental health patient to the extremely short stays of dental surgery and ear, nose, and throat procedures. These ALOS factors must be considered when forecasting future patient-day demand profiles.

Variations in ALOS can also be expected by unique age and sex cohorts. A profile of the total United States' ALOS suggests that males experience an ALOS of 8.1 days per admission, whereas females stay a shorter period at 7.3 days. Men who are 15 to 24 years old experience an ALOS of 5.9 days, which is different than women in the same age group, who stay only 4.3 days. However, if obstetrics is removed, lengths of stay by sex are closer (see table 25.)

Recognizing the dramatic variability in demand by age, sex, and specialty, shifts in any of these underlying variables could dramatically influence forecasted number of patient days and, therefore, forecasted gross revenue. Many hospitals in the United States, in fact, have made

Table 23 Average Length-of-Stay Comparative Analysis, 1984 versus 1983

Facility	1984	1983	Change
Memorial Hospital	6.94	7.51	0.57 days
All metropolitan hospitals	7.75	7.81	0.06 days

Source: PSRO data files for all Minneapolis-St. Paul hospitals

Table 24 Demand, by Patient Days, at Memorial Hospital

| | FY 1984 | | |
Specialty	Average Length of Stay	Patient Days	Distribution, %
Cardiology	7.6	3,844	4.8
Medicine	5.7	8,001	9.9
Surgery	7.7	9,110	11.3
Obstetrics	3.3	7,056	8.8
Gynecology	4.6	2,622	3.3
Urology	5.3	2,888	3.6
Orthopedics	7.1	6,134	7.6
Neurology	7.6	2,992	3.7
Dental surgery	1.7	39	0.01
Otorhinolaryngology	2.2	622	0.77
Ophthalmology	3.8	661	0.82
Mental health	17.0	14,667	17.8
Chemical dependency	16.8	10,798	13.4
Pediatrics	3.2	5,096	6.3
Newborn	3.3	5,977	7.4
Total	5.9	80,507	100.0

Source: Memorial Hospital medical records

errors in this regard. They have assumed erroneously that past demand would extend into the future because they anticipated increases in admissions, but failed to anticipate declines in ALOS adequately. In many markets, the declines in ALOS have been greater than the increases in admissions per thousand. Therefore, many hospitals have overanticipated the demand measured in patient days for several inpatient lines of business.

From a marketing and planning perspective, it is important to emphasize again the implications that changes in case mix can have on future revenue forecasts. And, expected shifts in case mix caused by changes in services or medical staff composition, marketing effectiveness, or competitive positioning for any line of business could materially alter a hospital's ALOS profile and, therefore, dramatically influence its patient-day and revenue potential.

Process

ALOS can be calculated by analyzing case information from the hospital medical record department, as well as similar information on all patients for all hospitals in the market area. Patient origin studies rely-

Table 25 U.S. Hospital Profile of
Average Length of Stay, by Age and Sex

Age and Sex Group	Average Length of Stay
Male	
Under 1	5.9
1–4	3.9
5–14	4.1
15–24	5.9
25–34	6.5
35–44	7.3
45–54	8.3
55–64	9.3
65–74	10.9
75+	12.0
Subtotal	8.1
Female	
Under 1	6.2
1–4	3.9
5–14	4.4
15–24	4.3
25–34	5.0
35–44	6.6
45–54	8.0
55–64	9.6
65–74	11.0
75+	12.1
Subtotal	7.3
Total	7.7

Source: U.S. Department of Health and Human
Services (actual 1980 data, not adjusted)

ing on samples of discharge abstracts and data tapes from PROs also
provide useful data for this purpose. It is important that the ALOS
assumptions used in the forecasting process be unique to the hospital
and not rely blindly on national or regional averages. Because ALOS
for a hospital is related to the unique case mix and practice style of its
medical staff, the ALOS by various specialties and certainly for the average admission, therefore, must be carefully developed using historical
information from within the hospital.

The ALOS for each service or specialty for the past three years can
be obtained by analyzing the medical records. This three-year trend will

indicate what assumptions should be made about the future direction and degree of change in the ALOS.

Forecasts of ALOS are influenced by the style of practice of the medical staff, which is in turn influenced by prevailing patterns of physician practice in the market area. Therefore, forecasts of ALOS should be tempered by an assessment of the overall trend of ALOS for the entire market area.

Issues

The calculation of ALOS is relatively straightforward and is used on an ongoing basis by the medical record department. The principal objective in the development of ALOS forecasts is not so much to evaluate historical experience, but to anticipate future shifts in the case mix of the various lines of business and to anticipate how low the ALOS will go during the 1980s as a result of changes in third-party reimbursement, the attitudes of medical school graduates, and advances in medical technology. In the past, many medical practitioners believed it was unlikely that the average community hospital would experience an ALOS less than 7 to 8 days. Many hospitals with a relatively standard case mix are now experiencing ALOS ranging as low as 4.5 days to 5.5 days.

Hospitals located in competitive environments within which HMOs and private utilization review for employers are established anticipate continuing pressure to reduce ALOS for most lines of business.

Data

The principal source of data for determining ALOS profiles is the medical record department. This can either be done on a sampling basis or by analysis of a full year's statistical base. The following additional data sources should be consulted as necessary:
- Reports from a patient discharge abstracting service
- Local PRO
- Local hospital planning organization
- *AHA Guide to the Health Care Field* and statistical reports
- U.S. Department of Health and Human Services

Stage 8: Forecasting Patient Days Used for Each Inpatient Service

Definitions

A *patient day* is a 24-hour period in which the customer, the patient, receives services rendered by hospital medical staff and employees. Patient days represent a critical building block for forecasting revenue and certain ancillary work loads, as well as for determining bed-need requirements for areawide planning purposes.

Patient days per thousand have been generally stable in the United States. However, many communities are now experiencing drops in the number of patient days per thousand as a result of public pressure to reduce the number of admissions per thousand and the ALOS, technology advances that allow more procedures to be done safely on an outpatient basis and patients to leave the hospital sooner, and economic pressure from insurance companies and HMOs to reduce demand for inpatient services.

Process

The process for forecasting patient days is straightforward and can be accomplished in three basic ways: the average length of stay times admissions method, the patient days per thousand method, and the specialty-specific method.

Average length of stay times admissions method. With this method, ALOS assumptions are multiplied by the projected number of admissions. For Memorial Hospital, the 14,927 admissions expected to occur in 1989 multiplied by an ALOS of 6.15 yields a forecast of 91,829 patient days. The number of patient days by specialty is calculated in a similar manner to illustrate the anticipated case mix for Memorial's various lines of business in 1989 (see table 26).

Examining Memorial's case mix suggests that in 1989 approximately 16,966 patient days or 18.5 percent of the hospital's demand is associated with mental health services. This line of business is expected to be challenged by third-party reimbursement sources during the 1980s. Substantial pressure will be exerted to meet the needs of these patients on a less expensive, outpatient basis and, for those admitted to the hospital, to shorten ALOS. The assumption that the ALOS in 1984 will remain constant through 1989 may, therefore, be dangerous to Memorial's financial planning. If during this five-year period, public pressure causes a 20 percent drop in the ALOS for mental health, Memorial Hospital would experience a traumatic drop in its total number of expected patient days and revenue in 1989.

Patient days per thousand method. With this method, historical patient days per thousand use rates are calculated and then used in conjunction with future population profile forecasts.

With respect to the U.S. population, the ALOS by age and sex multiplied by the number of admissions expected for each age and sex cohort

Table 26 Demand Measured in Patient Days
at Memorial Hospital, 1989

Specialty	Average Length of Stay, FY 1984	Admissions, 1989	Days, 1989*
Cardiology	7.6	582	4,423
Medicine	5.7	1,596	9,097
Surgery	7.7	1,358	10,457
Obstetrics	3.3	2,461	8,121
Gynecology	4.6	655	3,013
Urology	5.3	626	3,318
Orthopedics	7.1	1,000	7,100
Neurology	7.6	448	3,405
Dental surgery	1.7	30	51
Otorhinolaryngology	2.2	328	722
Ophthalmology	3.8	209	794
Mental health	17.0	998	16,966
Chemical dependency	16.8	685	11,508
Pediatrics	3.2	1,848	5,914
Newborn	3.3	2,103	6,940
Total	6.15	14,927	91,829

*Average length of stay × admissions = forecasted demand in days.

yields a total of 284,403,000 patient days (see table 27). However, males experience only 1,121 patient days per thousand, and females, 1,431, although the national average use rate is 1,280. These particular use rates vary significantly by age and by region of the United States. In addition, population groups that are enrolled in HMOs are experiencing anywhere from 450 to 650 patient days per thousand enrollees. As the HMO movement continues to expand in the United States, the number of patient days per thousand is expected to decrease. Therefore, the growing presence of HMOs in Memorial Hospital's market area will be a significant factor in the hospital's future demands.

Specialty-specific method. This method is based on forecasted admissions for each specialty, which are multiplied by the ALOS for each specialty. The general formula follows:

$Specialty_1$ admissions $\times$ $ALOS_1$ = Patient days$_1$
$Specialty_2$ admissions $\times$ $ALOS_2$ = Patient days$_2$
$Specialty_3$ admissions $\times$ $ALOS_3$ = Patient days$_3$

Patient days$_1$ + patient days$_2$ + patient days$_3$ = Total patient days

Table 27 U.S. Population Patient Day per 1,000 Use Rate

Age and Sex Group	Patient Days (thousands)	Days per 1,000
Male		
Under 1	2,467	
1–4	2,560	
5–14	4,201	
15–24	9,857	
25–34	10,760	
35–44	11,158	
45–54	14,772	
55–64	20,970	
65–74	24,193	
75+	20,429	
Subtotal	121,367	1,121
Female		
Under 1	1,852	
1–4	1,863	
5–14	3,602	
15–24	17,719	
25–34	22,119	
35–44	15,703	
45–54	17,815	
55–64	22,452	
65–74	26,562	
75+	33,350	
Subtotal	163,037	1,431
Total		
Under 1	4,318	1,241
1–4	4,423	353
5–14	7,802	230
15–24	27,576	664
25–34	32,879	909
35–44	26,862	104
45–54	32,587	1,436
55–64	43,421	2,048
65–74	50,756	3,276
75+	53,779	5,701
Total	284,403	1,280
Total patient days per 1,000		1,280

Source: Consultant report from Planmetrics, Chicago (actual 1980 data, not adjusted)

Issues

In the calculation of patient days during the forecasting process, attention must be given to assumptions made about ALOS for specific types of admissions. The above equations demonstrate substantial variability in ALOS by specialty and age and, to a lesser extent, sex. Simple extrapolation of ALOS for the average type of admission is therefore dangerous because of the important role that patient days play in determining aggregate hospital revenue.

Although the forecasts of future ALOS should be geared principally by a hospital's own historical experience and unique number and philosophies of its medical staff, forecasts must also be tempered by the prevailing trends within the market area.

Data

Principal information necessary to the base-case forecast of patient days is derived from data outputs in stage 6 and stage 7. If the patient day per thousand method is chosen to determine future patient days, these specialty-specific techniques should be used only as a method of validating the forecasts generated by the process described in stage 8.

Stage 9: Forecasting Ancillary Department Work-Load Volumes

Definitions

Ancillary departments that function as hospital revenue centers provide units of service that represent measurements of demand for those particular lines of business. These demand profiles usually are measured in numbers of tests or procedures. As hospitals treat patients who are more acutely ill and as pressures to reduce the ALOS continue, the trend in the United States is for the intensity of both diagnostic and therapeutic ancillary services to increase on a per admission basis. Memorial Hospital's work-load ratios vary dramatically among departments, and the ancillary work-load ratios have been changing during the past several years (see table 28). For example, the number of surgical procedures for medical and surgical inpatients decreased from .643 procedures per patient in 1980 to .600 procedures per patient in 1984. Radiology procedures per patient were 2.25 in 1980 and 2.09 in 1984, whereas respiratory therapy procedures increased from 2.03 in 1980 to 4.70 in 1984. In many of these ancillary lines of business, the trend has been for an increasing proportion of the work load to be performed on outpatients.

Table 28 Trends in Ancillary Work-Load Ratios at Memorial Hospital

Ancillary Department	1980	1981	1982	1983	1984
Operating room					
Procedures per medical-surgical-pediatric inpatient	.643	.649	.622	.628	.600
OP % of total	9.96	13.5	13.0	22.7	24.5
Radiology					
Procedures per patient	2.255	2.133	2.191	2.133	2.090
OP % of total	32.1	35.0	36.3	36.2	38.2
Nuclear medicine					
Procedures per patient	.065	.055	.052	.068	.078
OP % of total	32.7	47.4	53.7	53.9	56.1
Clinical laboratory					
Procedures per patient	11.15	10.50	10.87	10.83	10.83
OP % of total	15.1	16.3	17.1	17.7	17.5
Physical therapy					
Procedures per medical-surgical patient	.880	1.161	1.473	1.615	1.545
OP % of total	47.5	44.9	49.8	58.8	59.0
Occupational therapy					
Cardiac procedures per medical-pediatric care patient				1.05	1.50
OP % of total				3.07	25.4
General procedures per medical-surgical patient				.28	.28
OP % of total				11.3	11.6
Respiratory therapy					
Procedures per medical-surgical patient	2.03	2.18	4.88	4.43	4.70
OP % of total	2.62	1.92	6.59	7.08	6.74
EMG					
Procedures per patient	.015	.013	.013	.018	.016
OP % of total	47.1	49.4	63.7	59.5	71.3
EEG					
Procedures per patient	.033	.028	.027	.036	.038
OP % of total	33.7	35.1	30.5	25.6	29.1
EKG					
Procedures per patient	.563	.513	.561	.605	.606
OP % of total	9.7	11.4	12.5	14.8	15.2
Emergencies					
Visits per 1,000	116.07	117.63	124.10	124.11	127.15
Admission % of total	13.82	16.02	17.09	16.02	15.84

Source: Memorial Hospital medical records and billing records

Process

Ancillary utilization is a function of admissions and visits. The definition of the number of units expected to be consumed within each of the ancillary lines of business can be determined by first calculating historical ancillary work-load ratios and then multiplying these by forecasted numbers of admissions. Historical ancillary workload ratios can be generated by an evaluation of either medical record discharge information files or billing data tapes.

Forecasting future work loads is a straightforward process of multiplying defined ratios by forecasted admissions (or visits) of various services or specialties. For example, at Memorial Hospital in 1984 the workload ratio for operating room procedures per admission was 0.6 per admission (see table 29). Given the fact that 11,141 medical and surgical admissions are expected in 1989, 6,685 surgical procedures are projected for 1989. These ancillary department work-load volumes are predicated on the assumption that the work-load ratio of 1984 would remain constant until 1989 and that there would not be a significant shift in case mix.

Case-mix considerations are important because the consumption of ancillary department units of service varies by type of admission. If

Table 29 Forecasted Work-Load Volumes for Key Ancillary Services at Memorial Hospital

Ancillary Services	Work-Load Ratio per Admission, 1984	1989	
		Estimated Admissions*	Estimated Work-Load Volumes
Operating room	0.600	11,141	6,685
Radiology	2.090	12,824	26,802
Nuclear medicine	0.078	12,824	1,000
Clinical laboratory	10.830	12,824	138,884
Physical therapy	1.545	11,141	17,213
Occupational therapy			
cardiac	1.500	11,141	16,712
general	0.280	11,141	3,119
Respiratory therapy	4.700	11,141	52,363
EMG	0.016	12,824	205
EEG	0.038	12,824	487
EKG	0.606	12,824	7,771

*Medical and surgical patients = 11,141, excluding mental health, chemical dependency, and newborns. All patients = 14,927; less 2,103 newborns = 12,824.

Memorial Hospital were to experience a dramatic increase in the number of cardiology admissions, the average number of surgical procedures per typical admission would also have to be adjusted upward. There is a dramatic variation in ancillary use ratios for certain types of specialty admissions (see table 30).

Table 30 Variable Ratios of Ancillary SBU Demand, by Specialty

Ancillary	Demand Ratio per Admission		
Service (SBU)	Neurology	Oncology	Cardiology
Laboratory tests	8.22	18.58	16.67
Pharmacy prescriptions	8.08	17.98	10.23
Radiology	2.08	2.62	2.72
Physical therapy	1.69	0.42	0.15
Operating room procedures	0.40	0.90	0.02

Application of this forecasting approach yields work-load volumes that are of critical importance to subsequent planning and resource allocations. With a forecast of department workloads, standard ratios of departmental square footage can be determined and, therefore, facility parameters defined. With forecasts of ancillary department volumes, revenue and operating cost forecasts also can be developed. The hospital management group can thereby come to realize the importance of forecasting demand because of its direct relationship with planning for human resources, supply consumption, space requirements, revenue, and operating cost predictions. Hospital demand forecasting is a critical element in all facets of hospital planning and marketing. Forecasting tools and data bases are essential for the development and maintenance of integrated planning systems throughout a hospital.

Issues

Calculation of ancillary work-load volumes is not difficult, given the availability of statistical information from a hospital's routine medical records and billing data systems. An analysis of the medical record files or data tapes can be conducted for one year, or sampling methodologies can be used. However, hospital information systems do not always facilitate an easy linkage between the medical record data systems and the billing and financial data systems. It is essential to facilitate an easy integration of these systems because the billing and financial systems frequently have units of service and revenues per unit of service for aggregate and specialty admissions. These ancillary department volumes usually do not appear within the medical record system. To integrate a particular patient's ancillary department consumption and medical record history with respect to certain demographic features and diagnosis factors requires that the two data systems be manually or automatically linked. The critical element to the integration of these data systems is the assignment of a common patient identification number that appears on the patient's medical record and bill. Computer matching of these data files is desirable, but may result in the investment of substantial time and money.

The increasingly competitive environment not only will force hospitals to rely more heavily on prospectively negotiated budgets and case-mix payment, but also will make such investments essential.

An additional issue relates to the accuracy of extrapolating past utilization ratios into the future. Significant shifts in case mix or technology advances may materially alter these ancillary work-load ratios. A hospital's forecasting process must acknowledge this possibility throughout the forecasting process.

Data

As has previously been identified, data for accomplishing stage 9 activities are available within a hospital's medical record and billing systems. Although these data are available, they may not be easily accessible unless the hospital has faced the challenge of integrating the medical record and billing systems.

Summary

Chapter 3 has introduced the concepts and practice of hospital demand forecasting, using the experiences of a 277-bed general acute care community hospital to illustrate the concepts, strategies, and calculations of various stages of the demand forecasting process. A nine-stage process has been recommended: It begins with forecasts of population and use rates and builds from there through market share to ancillary department work volume. The concentration of this model upon population and market share information demonstrates the emphasis on population-based planning and market-based forecasting. The calculations contained in this chapter show how a base-case demand for a hospital's several lines of business can be developed. This base-case demand forecast is only a starting point for subsequent planning analyses, market research, and additional forecasting activities. The nature of a hospital's approach to refining and updating this base case are discussed in the next chapter.

Chapter 4

Scenario Development: The Use of Judgment to Move Beyond the Base Case

Scenario development enables hospital managers to: (1) define alternate future environments within which they can evaluate implications of the base-case demand forecast for hospital operations, (2) alter the base-case forecast by challenging the underlying assumptions upon which the base-case forecast has been developed, and (3) evaluate the impact that refinements to the demand forecast will have on future hospital operations.

This chapter examines alternate ways to develop future scenarios and the role scenario development can play in refining the base-case forecast. The use of judgment in forecasting is examined in the process of environmental scanning, scenario development techniques, and implications of scenario development in future demand forecasts at Memorial Hospital.

As described in the previous chapter, the base-case forecast for a given hospital is generated under the presumption that the past utilization experiences for hospitals within that marketplace will remain virtually constant in the future, as will this particular hospital's share of the market's aggregate demand for hospital services. The only factors expected to change in the future are the service area's unique demographic profile measured by the number of persons by age and sex cohort.

However, in and of itself, the base-case forecast is inadequate input for the hospital's strategic planning and market planning processes. The complexity and rapidly changing nature of the several factors that influence capital demand indicate that hospital managers would not be prudent to base operational actions only upon forecasted demand. The forces that generated past utilization experiences are unlikely to exist in the same form and in the same degree in the future. Therefore, hospital managers should use the base-case only *as a starting point for its planning process* and factor in additional information and assumptions regarding the future operating environment. The process of evaluating major trends and developments in the external operating environment of a hospital and its market area is called *environmental scanning*.

Environmental Scanning

Environmental scanning is the process of assessing the external environment within which a particular industry or corporation is operating. It attempts to identify and interpret major factors that influence the hospital's operations in terms of utilization, technology, practice of medicine, legislation, and so forth. Environmental scanning came into its own as a concept during the 1970s when several industries attempted to refine their corporate planning processes.

Developing explicit scenarios about the future operating environment is an important mechanism that ensures judgment is used in the planning and forecasting process. (See appendix D for an executive summary of an environmental assessment report for a multihospital system.) An eight-step process is required for the structured application of judgment in the demand forecasting process (see figure 7). An important component of this process is developing a structured approach to evaluate potential changes in demand-influencing factors (the third step in environmental scanning): it encourages hospital managers to establish work sheets that identify those factors expected to have the most substantial impact on hospital demand. A worksheet can be used to calculate changes in the base-case forecast of aggregate demand within a given market area by evaluating the potential implications of changes in key factors and how these might affect the admission rates per thousand, the ALOS per admission, visits per thousand, and admissions for ancillary department units (see figure 8). Work sheets should be used for each of the hospital's principal programs or lines of business.

Environmental scanning should therefore be viewed as a process of evaluating trends in the various demand-influencing factors. This scanning should be done prior to the utilization of worksheets. Environ-

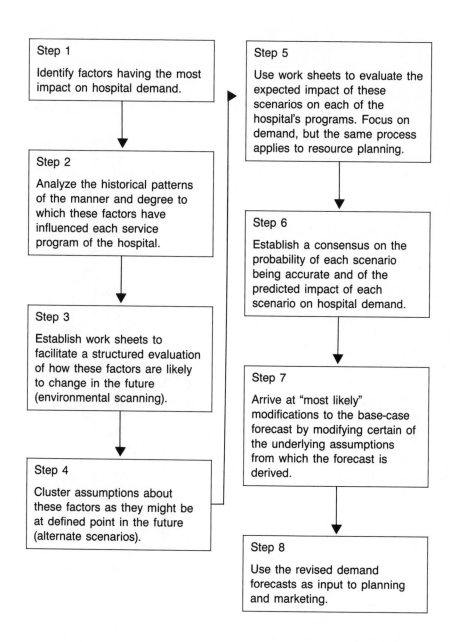

Step 1

Identify factors having the most impact on hospital demand.

Step 2

Analyze the historical patterns of the manner and degree to which these factors have influenced each service program of the hospital.

Step 3

Establish work sheets to facilitate a structured evaluation of how these factors are likely to change in the future (environmental scanning).

Step 4

Cluster assumptions about these factors as they might be at defined point in the future (alternate scenarios).

Step 5

Use work sheets to evaluate the expected impact of these scenarios on each of the hospital's programs. Focus on demand, but the same process applies to resource planning.

Step 6

Establish a consensus on the probability of each scenario being accurate and of the predicted impact of each scenario on hospital demand.

Step 7

Arrive at "most likely" modifications to the base-case forecast by modifying certain of the underlying assumptions from which the forecast is derived.

Step 8

Use the revised demand forecasts as input to planning and marketing.

Figure 7 Conceptual overview of attempt to inject judgment into the demand forecasting process

Base-Case Use Rate Assumptions, by Specialty	Expected Impact on Use Rates					Overall Expected Direction of Change within Three Years			Overall Degree of Change, %
	Morbidity in Area	New Technology	New Treatments	New Reimbursement	Other	Up	Down	Same	
Ophthalmology									
Orthopedics									
Urology									
General medicine									
Pediatrics									
Obstetrics									
Gynecology									
Psychiatry									
Chemical dependency									
General surgery									
Oral surgery									
Oncology									
Cardiology									
Neurology									
Emergency									
Other									

Figure 8 Work sheet to probe future use rates

Existing Base-Case Market Share, by Specialty	Expected Influence on Market Share				Expected Overall Direction of Change			Expected Degree of Change, %
	New Physicians on Staff	Action of Competitors	New Public Relations Efforts	Other	Up	Down	Same	
Ophthalmology								
Orthopedics								
Urology								
General medicine								
Pediatrics								
Obstetrics								
Gynecology								
Psychiatry								
Chemical dependency								
General surgery								
Oral surgery								
Oncology								
Cardiology								
Neurology								
Emergency								
Other								

Figure 9 Work sheet on market share

mental scanning will assist those who use the work sheets to better understand the anticipated trends within the demand-influencing factors and to provide a context in which to judge the implications of the trends on hospital demand.

The American Hospital Association, in its publication *Environmental Assessment of the Hospital Industry, 1979,* examined a number of forces influencing the U.S. hospital industry and identified the anticipated implication of those forces on future hospital operations. The following major areas were identified:

- Changes in demographic patterns and patient use characteristics within the United States
- Industry composition and the structure of changing interactions with other health providers
- Financing of hospital services and shifts in third-party payment
- Changing regulations, legislation, and litigation
- Human resources and the availability of workers to hospitals
- The scope and nature of hospital services offered within the hospital's portfolio of health programs
- The organization of hospitals in terms of governance, management, and medical staff

The Hospital Research and Educational Trust, a research and development affiliate of the American Hospital Association, has published an update of this assessment titled *Environmental Assessment, 1984.* The American Hospital Association initiated this environmental scan on the premise that sound strategic planning for any organization must be based on a systematic examination of the environment that organization is and will be facing. This examination includes an interpretation of potential implications of trends in those factors that influence demand and future operations of hospitals. Environmental scanning, therefore, represents an opportunity for hospital managers to inject judgment into the forecasting and planning processes. The challenge is to ensure that this injection of judgment is done in a sufficiently structured and explicit manner.

Environmental scanning is also an essential process used to determine anticipated shifts in those factors that influence a hospital's particular market share within the aggregate demand for hospital services in the market area. Hospital managers can also use a work sheet to test the future implications of trend factors that are important to a hospital's ability to expand its market share for a specific service (see figure 9).

There is nothing particularly magic about the concept of environmental scanning or the use of worksheets in hospital strategic planning and marketing activities. Environmental scanning parallels much of hospital planning's traditional examination of external forces that operate in the hospital's service area or the hospital industry. Environmental scanning as a concept, however, assists hospital managers improve their external evaluation process by encouraging a more explicit and rigorous examination of a wide range of factors that influence not only aggregate demand for hospital services, but also the potential market share of that aggregate demand. The work sheets simply assist hospital managers to avoid overlooking or failing to take certain factors seriously enough in the planning processes.

How can a hospital improve its environmental scanning activities? A number of resources are available for hospital managers to improve the scope and sophistication of their environmental scanning techniques. An important principle is to rely as much as possible on existing studies and research efforts. Borrowing from others will avoid reinventing the wheel or the unnecessary expenditure of scarce time and money from the hospital's planning and marketing efforts. The following sources provide data and data analyses for this purpose:

- Local, state, and regional economic planning and development councils
- Local and regional chambers of commerce
- State health planning and demographers' offices
- Local and state hospital associations
- Regional and state health planning agencies
- Economic research departments of local universities and colleges
- Faculty of graduate programs in hospital and health care administration
- Health care workers education programs
- Professional associations representing various hospital management perspectives
- Research staff from health and social welfare committees of the state legislature and of the U.S. Congress
- Research staff from the U.S. Department of Health and Human Services, in particular the Health Care Financing Administration, National Center for Health Services Research and Development, the National Center for Health Statistics, and the Bureau for Health Planning

A number of state hospital associations and multihospital systems currently are conducting their own environmental assessment activities, which also may be used to stimulate and shape an individual hospital's environmental scanning activities.

After analyzing the direction and degree of change in the major factors that influence hospital demand, the challenge is to forecast the shifts in the future demand for a hospital's services these trends will create. The injection of judgment for interpreting shifts in hospital demand should be made on as small a unit of demand as possible, for example, cardiology admissions. In addition, it should involve alternative processes for distilling the opinions of diverse groups of planning participants with respect to the direction, degree, and impact of shifts in future hospital demand. Achieving a consensus about the implications on demand for units of service is not easy, and, therefore, hospital managers should become more familiar with group planning techniques. These techniques can be used to develop alternative scenarios of the future operating environment, as well as to predict the effect these scenarios will have on the hospital's operations.

Scenario Development

As a result of environmental scanning, hospital staff members are better informed to develop alternate future scenarios for hospital market areas. *Scenarios* are defined simply as predictions about a future environment, clustering and varying assumptions about key elements of a hospital's operating environment in unique ways.

This cluster of assumptions is stated in straightforward terms for a defined point in the future. Two or three alternate scenarios frequently are developed to reflect a range of assumptions for each factor influencing the hospital's future demand. (See appendix D for an illustration of how alternate future scenarios have been used within the hospital sector.)

The eight-step approach for applying judgment in demand forecasting (see figure 7) identifies an important challenge for hospital managers: to understand the probability of future demand forecasts in order to reflect future reality accurately. This presumes that the likelihood of an individual's prediction being accurate probably is less than the accuracy of a consensus reached by a large group of experts. There are two general techniques available that will facilitate reaching a group consensus regarding the future, that is, to challenge or modify the base-case forecast: brainstorming and Delphi panel.

Brainstorming

The simplest methodology for reaching group consensus during forecasting and planning is brainstorming. This technique requires a group of knowledgeable persons familiar with the hospital, its service area, and its competitive posture gathering to evaluate the trends expected to influence aggregate market demand, the factors that could influence the hospital's share of this market, and the impact of these trends on the future demand of the hospital's services.

A group facilitator frequently records the group's ideas in a random list and assists the group in reaching conclusions about future demand. Work sheets, such as those previously described, can be employed to stimulate and to guide such brainstorming sessions. In general, the brainstorming approach occurs within one or two group meetings and results in a written document summarizing the findings and conclusions reached during the group discussion. The advantage of the brainstorming approach is its simplicity and low cost. Because brainstorming sessions frequently include persons from within the hospital organization, it has the added advantage of establishing internal understanding of the conclusions reached during the group's deliberations.

The brainstorming approach, however, has a number of disadvantages associated with its simplicity:

- Heavy reliance on hospital staff may result in a group with limited perspectives. Without a full range of perspectives, potential shifts in the factors influencing hospital demand may not be adequately evaluated. This technique also can result in a lack of candor from staff members who may have a vested interest in predicting an inaccurate demand pattern for their areas of responsibility.
- The general tendency to complete the brainstorming session within one or two group meetings suggests that the evaluation and thought processes of the individual members of the group may be too shallow to rigorously challenge and think through the long-range implications of complicated demand-influencing factors.
- The ultimate validity and reliability of conclusions reached in the brainstorming session may be unnecessarily dependent on the skills and biases of the group facilitator, who leads the brainstorming session.

Although the brainstorming session has the appeal of applying judgment to the forecasting process in a relatively short and inexpensive manner, the influence of these disadvantages may not yield the most accurate modifications of the base-case forecast.

The Delphi Technique

Corporations and hospitals are relying increasingly on a specialized technique called the Delphi technique for getting a diverse group of individuals to reach a consensus. A panel of recognized experts representing many facets of a hospital's operations is assembled. For example, a physician for each specialty, financial staff, third-party reimbursers, regional economic planners, health systems agency staff, and prominent regional medical researchers are often included in Delphi panels. These panelists are oriented to their role and the process by mail or in a retreat setting. Hospital managers distribute the following information to focus the panel's deliberations, meanwhile being careful not to color interpretations:

- Work sheets that identify which units of demand will be forecasted and which demand factors are to be assessed (see figures 8 and 9).
- The base-case forecast and the underlying assumptions upon which it has been derived
- The environmental scanning report, which documents major trends of the factors that influence future demand

Members of the panel are asked individually to assess the factors that influence hospital demand and to rate the probability or significance of these factors. Opinions are shared by means of structured questionnaires or worksheets, which are completed at least two times in at least two stages.

During the first stage, the Delphi panelists individually and anonymously complete the work sheets to identify the specific direction and the degree of change they believe hospital demand will take at some specified point in the future (usually five years). The degree of change is frequently stated in terms of a percentage. For example, a panel member might indicate that five years from now oncology admissions per thousand population will increase by five percent. Responses to the questionnaire or worksheets are collected and summarized to achieve an average response pattern for the group. The summary responses are given to each member of the panel as input for subsequent deliberations. During the second stage, the panel members re-examine their previous responses in light of the combined summary of all the other panelists and are given the opportunity to modify their previous responses if appropriate. The second stage is concluded when a reasonable consensus is reached about what factors influence demand and when the panel members have confidence in their conclusions.

Although some applications of the Delphi technique involve three and four iterations of this process, the cost effectiveness generally is maximized with the two-stage approach.

Following the identification of those factors judged to have the most impact on future hospital demand, the Delphi technique also can be applied to anticipate the exact direction and degree to which the base-case forecast will be changed as a result of trends in the demand-influencing factors.

As a result of this structured evaluation of the potential demand for each unit of service, hospital managers are able to determine the need for and the nature of modifications to the base-case forecast. The modifications are implemented by altering the underlying assumptions used to derive this forecast. It is conceivable that a Delphi panel would suggest that aggregate hospital demand in a given service area may decline for many inpatient programs and increase for several outpatient programs. However, the panel might also suggest that an individual hospital's share of this forecasted aggregate demand may go up in some programs and down in others, based upon the panel members' consensus about shifts in the hospital's competitive posture, changing consumer preferences, and utilization patterns.

The Delphi technique, therefore, represents a useful tool for establishing alternate future scenarios of the operating environment within which the hospital intends to compete for demand, and also for reaching a group consensus on the implications, within each scenario, of the various forces of hospital demand.

If three scenarios are developed, there are three new forecasts of future hospital demand to compare. Comparison of these three forecasts to the base-case forecast enables hospital managers to judge whether additional management actions and initiatives to expand market share are needed; to anticipate whether additional resources, such as manpower, facilities, equipment, and supplies are needed; and to assess the potential impact of these alternative futures on internal hospital operating policies and procedures. Scenario development becomes an essential step early in the hospital strategic planning process, and the use of the Delphi technique to establish these scenarios and test the impact of these alternative futures provides important input to a hospital's subsequent planning. The following areas, in particular, benefit from scenario development:

- Marketing strategies
- Certificate-of-need and capital expenditure planning
- Human resources planning
- Overall budgeting and financial planning activities

Modification of Memorial Hospital's Base-Case Forecast

Members of the Memorial Hospital management staff conducted special studies of operating trends in the market area in an attempt to anticipate shifts in the underlying assumptions driving the hospital's future demand. Work sheets were used to gauge the potential effect of changes in basic demand-influencing factors on utilization rates, market share, and ALOS. The overall conclusion reached was that most of the demand-influencing factors would change substantially (see table 31). Memorial Hospital anticipated that several of the specialty use rates would go up as a result of modest increases in the elderly population. Demand, as

Table 31 Percent Shift in Demand Assumptions from the Base Case at Memorial Hospital*

Specialty	Use Rate	Market Share	Average Length of Stay	Intensity of Ancillaries
Oncology	10	7	(5)	5
Cardiology	5	6	(5)	5
Psychiatry	(25)	(15)	(25)	5
Chemical dependency	(30)	(15)	(40)	5
Ophthalmology	0	5	(5)	5
Otorhinolaryngology	(10)	0	2	5
Neurology	3	5	0	5
Orthopedics	5	5	(5)	5
Urology	(5)	5	5	5
Gynecology	(3)	5	0	5
Obstetrics	0	6	(5)	5
Pediatrics and pediatric medicine	(5)	0	0	5
General medical	2	7	(5)	5
General surgery	0	5	(5)	5

*Assumes change from 1984 to 1989, steady from 1989 to 1994.

measured by utilization rates, however, was expected to drop dramatically in psychiatry and chemical dependency, with more modest decreases in specialties in which there have been technological advances to enable more outpatient activity.

With respect to market share, the planning participants at Memorial Hospital anticipated increases in most areas as a result of initiatives planned by hospital medical staff and managers for the next five years. The actions contemplated include promotional activities, physician recruitment, and the establishment of satellite facilities on the periphery of the hospital's service area.

The planning participants assumed a basic reduction in ALOS for most specialties. In addition, continued pressure from third-party payers and advances in technology were expected to reduce the number of inpatient procedures and the overall ALOS. Dramatic decreases were expected in the ALOS for psychiatry and mental health, whereas slight increases were forecasted for otorhinolaryngology and neurology patients under the presumption that once admitted, these patients would be at a higher acuity level and, therefore, would require additional time in the hospital.

Forecasting the future trend in utilization of various diagnostic and therapeutic ancillary services is difficult. Analysis of national trends suggests that the intensity of ancillary use per patient has been increasing steadily. The planning participants at Memorial Hospital accordingly assumed that, although this upward trend would continue, it would be constrained to approximately five percent from 1984 to 1989 and then would hold steady between 1989 and 1994.

Conclusions reached in all of these areas were open to challenge by all planning participants within Memorial Hospital and in its market area. Utilization of the work sheets to make these assumptions explicit guarded against extravagant or inappropriate new demand assumptions. As a result of these shifts in underlying assumptions for Memorial's demand, the forecasting process identified in chapter 2 should be reinitiated for Memorial Hospital. The following pages describe the results of applying this new set of assumptions to the base-case demand forecast at Memorial Hospital.

Adjusting Utilization Rates

Under the alternate scenario for the period 1984 to 1989, the use rate for cardiology patients, for example, is expected to increase by a factor of five percent (see table 32). With an original use rate of 11.36 admis-

Table 32 Adjusting the Use Rate with Judgment
about the Future Environment

Specialty	Prior Use Rate	Subjective % Adjustment, 1984 to 1989	1989 Forecasted Use Rate*
Cardiology	11.36	5	11.93
General medical and surgical and oncology	42.30	5	44.42
Obstetrics	13.90	—	13.90
Gynecology	4.47	(3)	4.34
Urology	4.74	(5)	4.50
Orthopedics	14.70	5	15.44
Neurology	2.66	3	2.74
Otorhinolaryngology	3.80	(10)	3.42
Ophthalmology	3.16	—	3.16
Mental health	6.04	(25)	4.53
Chemical dependency	3.94	(30)	2.76
Pediatrics	8.41	(5)	7.99
Newborns	11.67	—	11.67
Total	131.20		130.80

*Prior use rate × subjective adjustment = forecasted use rate.

sions per thousand, this adjustment would yield an anticipated 1984 to 1989 utilization rate of 11.93 admissions per thousand. Similarly, the original mental health utilization rate of 6.04 admissions per thousand is expected to be reduced to a use rate of 4.53 admissions per thousand. The overall utilization rate for the Memorial Hospital market area is reduced slightly from a use rate of 131.2 admissions per thousand in 1984 to an anticipated use rate of 130.8 in 1989.

Determining New Aggregate Admissions for the Market Area

The strategic planning process within Memorial Hospital led to the conclusion that the utilization rate for 1989 will hold relatively constant through the year 1994. Application of these utilization rates to the forecasted population at 1994 for Memorial Hospital's market area will yield new aggregate admissions for the market area (see table 33). For example, the utilization rate of 11.93 admissions per thousand in cardiology would yield 4,278 cardiology admissions for 1994. This aggregate number of admissions represents the total market for cardiology admissions within which Memorial and its medical staff will be competing. Similarly, the orthopedics use rate of 15.44 admissions per thousand sug-

Table 33 New Use Rates and Aggregate Admissions for the Service Area, by Specialty

Specialty	New Use Rates[a] for 1989	1994 Admissions for Service Area[b]
Cardiology	11.93	4,278
General medical and surgical and oncology	44.42	15,929
Obstetrics	13.90	4,984
Gynecology	4.34	1,556
Urology	4.50	1,614
Orthopedics	15.44	5,537
Neurology	2.74	983
Otorhinolaryngology	3.42	1,226
Ophthalmology	3.16	1,133
Mental health	4.53	1,624
Chemical dependency	2.76	990
Pediatrics	7.99	2,865
Newborns	11.67	4,185
Total	130.80	46,904

[a]From table 32.

[b]Based upon 1994 service area population of 358,590. Does not include admissions from outside the defined service area.

gests that in 1994, the market area would generate 5,537 orthopedic admissions. Applying the use rates of all specialties to the 1994 population forecasts would yield an aggregate market of 46,904 admissions.

Adjusting Market Share by Specialty Services

Making market share assumptions explicit by specialty enables all planning participants to understand the underlying assumptions for future demand forecasts and to take issue with these assumptions as necessary. Although Memorial Hospital experienced a 13 percent market share for all cardiology in its principal market area in 1984, the six percent adjustment increase would yield a 1989 market share of 13.8 percent (see table 34). However, the services in mental health and chemical dependency are forecasted to lose market share, resulting in a drop in chemical dependency from 44.2 percent to 37.6 percent during the five-year period. It is anticipated that this drop in market share will result in a loss of admissions from Memorial's hospital-based chemical dependency program to competing free-standing residential treatment centers that will be developed in the area. These market share increases represent a reversal in the downward slippage of market share

Table 34 New 1989 Market Share Profile at Memorial Hospital

Specialty	Market Share for 1984, %	Adjustment to Market Share, 1984-1989, %	Forecasted 1989 Market Share, %*
Cardiology	13.0	6	13.8
General medical and surgical and oncology	17.8	7	19.1
Obstetrics	44.9	6	47.6
Gynecology	37.2	5	39.1
Urology	33.5	5	35.2
Orthopedics	17.3	5	18.2
Neurology	42.7	5	44.8
Otorhinolaryngology	21.9	—	21.9
Ophthalmology	16.8	5	17.6
Mental health	42.0	(15)	35.7
Chemical dependency	44.2	(15)	37.6
Pediatrics	55.4	—	55.4
Newborns	45.7	6	48.4
Total	28.8		

*1984 forecasted market share × adjustment to market share from 1984 to 1989 = 1989 forecasted market share.

experienced by Memorial Hospital from 1982 to 1984 and will require major management action to ensure their happening.

Forecasting Future Admissions

The forecasted number of admissions that Memorial Hospital expects to experience in 1994 encompasses the assumptions that its market share will increase from 1984 to 1989 as previously mentioned and that this 1989 market share will hold constant to the year 1994 (see table 35). Application of these new assumptions in cardiology suggests that for the aggregate demand in the market area of 4,278 admissions, Memorial Hospital's market share of 13.8 percent would yield 590 cardiology admissions in 1994. Similarly, of the 5,537 total market for orthopedics, Memorial Hospital's 18.2 percent would yield 1,008 admissions in 1994. Decreases in market share forecasted for mental health and chemical dependency showed dramatic decreases in demand for these services in 1994. As a result of these new market share forecasts, Memorial Hospital is anticipating that its 1994 demand as measured in inpatient admissions will be 16,855 total admissions (see table 36).

Table 35 New 1994 Memorial Hospital Admissions

Specialty	Demand in Area	New 1989 Market Share Forecasts, %	1989 Admissions*
Cardiology	4,278	13.8	590
General medical and surgical and oncology	15,929	19.1	3,042
Obstetrics	4,984	47.6	2,372
Gynecology	1,556	39.1	608
Urology	1,614	35.2	568
Orthopedics	5,537	18.2	1,008
Neurology	983	44.8	440
Otorhinolaryngology	1,226	21.9	268
Ophthalmology	1,133	17.6	199
Mental health	1,624	35.7	580
Chemical dependency	990	37.6	372
Pediatrics	2,865	55.4	1,587
Newborns	4,185	48.4	2,026
Subtotal for principal market area	46,904		13,660
Other areas (17% of Memorial Hospital's total demand)			2,802
Total			16,462

*Demand × new 1989 market share forecasts = forecasted 1989 admissions.

Table 36 Memorial Hospital Admissions in 1989

Specialty	1984	1985	1986	1987	1988	1989	1990	1991	1992	1993	1994
Cardiology	526					618					710
General medical and surgical and oncology	2,699					3,180					3,661
Obstetrics	2,225					2,547					2,870
Gynecology	592					664					735
Urology	566					625					684
Orthopedics	904					1,059					1,214
Neurology	405					468					531
Otorhinolaryngology	297					310					323
Ophthalmology	189					215					241
Mental health	699					801					903
Chemical dependency	448					534					620
Pediatrics	1,659					1,786					1,912
Newborns	1,902					2,177					2,451
Total	13,111					14,984					16,855

Determining Demand for Target Year 1989

The planning participants at Memorial Hospital previously identified the year 1989 as their principal planning horizon. To forecast demand for its inpatient lines of business in 1989, two methodologies can be followed:

- The nine-stage forecasting process
- The straight-line extrapolation between actual demand in 1984 and forecasted demand in 1994

The lack of readily available population statistics relating to 1989 has caused Memorial Hospital managers to use the extrapolation technique between 1984 and 1994. The aggregate demand for Memorial in 1989 is therefore forecasted to be 14,986 patients (see table 37). Utilization of the straight-line extrapolation methodology has the potential for error if the growth rate of each specialty is not constant from 1984 to 1994. This potential error must be taken into consideration during subsequent planning and decision-making activities.

Table 37 New 1989 Average Length-of-Stay Forecast for Memorial Hospital

Specialty	Average Length of Stay, Days	Adjustment to Average Length of Stay, %	New 1989 Forecasted Average Length of Stay
Cardiology	7.6	(5)	7.2
Medicine	5.7	(5)	5.4
Surgery	7.7	(5)	7.3
Obstetrics	3.3	(5)	3.1
Gynecology	4.6	—	4.6
Urology	5.3	5	5.6
Orthopedics	7.1	(5)	6.7
Neurology	7.2	—	7.2
Dental surgery	1.2	—	1.2
Otorhinolaryngology	2.2	2	2.2
Ophthalmology	3.8	(5)	3.6
Mental health	17.0	(25)	12.8
Chemical dependency	16.8	(40)	10.1
Pediatrics	3.2	—	3.2
Newborn	3.3	—	3.3

Determining New Average Length-of-Stay Factors

The next step is to modify the base-case ALOS profile for each specialty (see table 37). Where the 1984 ALOS for cardiology was 7.6 days, the forecasted adjustment for a decrease of five percent yields a 1989 ALOS of 7.2 days. Similarly, orthopedic admissions drops from 7.1 days in 1984 to 6.7 days in 1989. Dramatic decreases in ALOS are forecasted to occur in mental health and chemical dependency, which drop from 17 days to 12.8 days and 16.8 days to 10.1 days, respectively.

Determining Patient Days

Adding the ALOS to the new scenario forecast of admissions enables planning participants to generate a forecast of new patient days (see table 38). The 618 cardiology admissions forecasted by Memorial Hospital multiplied by an expected ALOS of 7.2 days yields a forecast of 4,450 cardiology patient days in 1989. This same methodology is applied to all specialties and to the aggregate figures. The forecasted 1989 admissions of 14,986 yields 78,807 total patient days, for an ALOS of 5.3 days. The planning participants accordingly modified their future ALOS from 6.1 days to 5.3 days.

Table 38 New Patient Days at Memorial Hospital, 1989

Specialty	New Admissions	New Average Length of Stay	New Patient Days
Cardiology	618	7.2	4,450
General medical and surgical and oncology	3,182	6.1	19,410
Obstetrics	2,547	3.1	7,896
Gynecology	664	4.6	3,054
Urology	625	5.6	3,500
Orthopedics	1,059	6.7	7,095
Neurology	468	7.2	3,370
Otorhinolaryngology	310	2.3	713
Ophthalmology	215	3.6	774
Mental health	801	12.8	10,253
Chemical dependency	534	10.1	5,393
Pediatrics	1,786	3.2	5,715
Newborn	2,177	3.3	7,184
Total	14,986	5.3	78,807

As a result of reconsidering the underlying demand assumptions from the base case, the planning participants at Memorial Hospital forecasted a future demand for 78,807 days compared to an original base-case forecast of 91,829 days (see table 39). This is a 14.2 percent decrease in demand. If Memorial Hospital had conducted its resource allocation decisions under the assumption that there would be 91,829 days, but actually secured only 78,807, the amount of budgeted revenue would not have been achieved and the expenses would have been greater than they needed to be to respond to the demand. This situation demonstrates the importance not only of having accurate demand forecasts, but also of testing the assumptions of the base case with alternate scenarios of the future.

Table 39 Comparative Analysis of Patient Day Forecasts under Alternate Scenarios at Memorial Hospital, 1989

| Specialty | Alternate Scenarios | | |
	Base Case	New Case	Difference, %
Cardiology	4,423	4,450	0.6
General medical and surgical	19,605	19,410	(.99)
Obstetrics	8,121	7,896	(2.8)
Gynecology	3,013	3,054	1.36
Urology	3,318	3,500	5.5
Orthopedics	7,100	7,095	(.07)
Neurology	3,405	3,370	(1.03)
Otorhinolaryngology	722	713	(1.2)
Ophthalmology	794	774	(2.5)
Mental health	16,966	10,253	(39.6)
Chemical dependency	11,508	5,393	(53.1)
Pediatrics	5,914	5,715	(3.36)
Newborn	6,940	7,184	3.5
Total	91,829	78,807	(14.2)

As a result of testing new demand forecasts within alternate scenarios, the planning and marketing participants at Memorial Hospital are now faced with the challenge of initiating certain actions designed to achieve or exceed the forecasted demand numbers.

Determining New Ancillary Department Work-Load Volumes

Forecasting new ancillary department work-load volumes is a function of admissions and visits, similar to the process discussed in chapter 3.

Forecasting new work loads is a process of multiplying previously defined ratios by the number of forecasted new admissions (or visits) of various services or specialties. New ancillary department work-load volumes are, once again, predicated on the assumption that the work-load ratio of 1984 will remain constant until 1989 and that there will not be a significant shift in case mix. In the process of defining new work-load volume ratios, however, the hospital's management should give careful thought to the various trends or issues that may have a strong impact on ancillary department work-load volumes, including, but not limited to:
- New technology
- Changing reimbursement patterns
- Shortened length of stay and higher ancillary intensity
- Changing style of physician practice

Summary

Chapter 4 introduced the concepts of scenario development to move a hospital beyond the base case by using subjective inputs to the forecast. It provided the basis for "what-if" analysis, enabling the hospital to analyze the impact that refinements of the base case will have on future hospital operations.

The processes included environmental scanning, brainstorming, and the Delphi technique for the development of alternative future scenarios. The outcomes of these techniques were applied to the base-case forecast to arrive at alternative, more realistic scenarios for management to consider in planning for future demand.

Epilogue

This book has established the need for strengthened forecasting processes, development of the base case, and adjustment of the base case through the use of judgment in scenario development. Once the principles of this book have been applied, hospital managers will be able to modify the forecasting methods to develop alternative strategies to enhance utilization. Although this book has not dealt with the forecasting of outpatient utilization, the principles are the same.

Forecasts are an effective mechanism for accomplishing the following activities:

- Defining an institution's current market position
- Defining where an institutions demand should be in the future
- Forcing the use of judgment in defining future market positions
- Preparing for alternative reimbursement mechanisms
- Forcing or strengthening the link between financial and planning information systems
- Enhancing the potential for information sharing among local or areawide institutions
- Adjusting staff to demand
- Identifying weaknesses in existing strategy or potential new strategies to enhance market share and utilization

For these reasons, forecasting spans disciplines and provides key input into most phases of hospital operations. It is no longer an option, but an indispensable function of the hospital management process. It is also a function that requires eclectic methods, a mix of qualitative and quantitative techniques, and the insights and judgments of many disciplines.

Appendix A

Matching Population Data to Zip Code Areas

Although conceivably there are several ways to accomplish the task of matching the population data that may be available to a hospital to the appropriate zip code areas, all of them are complicated by the fact that more than 5,000 changes to zip code areas are made per year by local postmasters. The whole process of assigning zip codes is governed locally, and the boundaries and zip code areas are reassigned on a regular basis. However, the revisions to the zip code boundaries are generally minor and should have little effect on forecast data.

The larger problem actually is assigning the hospital's primary and secondary service areas to the appropriate zip code boundaries. In many communities, this is done by the chamber of commerce, city planning and development government bodies, health planning agencies, neighboring institutions, and other government and nongovernment bodies. If, however, these data are not readily available, several other sources exist, including Donnelly Marketing Services, Oakbrook, IL, and CACI, Inc., Los Angeles, CA:

Donnelly offers two fine software packages known as X-Census Plus and American Profile. The user has the option of actually subscribing to the service or requesting computer runs of areas. Maps with defined service areas can be contoured into zip code areas, census tracts, metropolitan statistical areas, and so forth. The zip code areas used by the Donnelly model are updated annually, and, therefore, information is current.

CACI, Inc. offers software packages that are similar to those described above. They are called Site, Site II, and Potential. They have similar benefits to those described above, however, the data are not updated as regularly and the firm does not do an annual revision by zip code areas. The model can be run from maps.

Should these methods prove unworkable for a hospital's needs, it is likely that assistance can be obtained from the American Hospital Association or from the information systems or planning divisions of many multihospital systems.

Sample Market Research Instrument

The Medical Center Community Health Care Survey

Please circle your response:

1. How long has it been since you or someone else in your family stayed overnight in a hospital?
   - a. Less than one year
   - b. One to three years
   - c. More than three years
   - d. Never
   - e. Do not know

2. Thinking of the most recent stay someone in your household had at a hospital, were you in the hospital, or was it another family member?
   - a. You
   - b. Other family member

3. What hospital was it that you/your family member stayed in last?

   _____

4. Please circle the response that best describes why you/your family member was in the hospital:
   - a. Tests/exam (X-ray/lab only)
   - b. To have a baby
   - c. Surgery
   - d. Illness not requiring surgery
   - e. Pediatric care
   - f. Emergency
   - g. Chemical dependency
   - h. Mental health
   - i. Other (specify): _____

5. Who chose the hospital?
   a. My physician   b. I did   c. Both my physician and I
   d. Other (please specify): _____

6. Thinking back to that last hospital stay, please rate the following services:

		Excellent	Good	Fair	Poor	Do Not Know
a.	Cleanliness	1	2	3	4	5
b.	Quality of physician care	1	2	3	4	5
c.	Nursing care	1	2	3	4	5
d.	Quality of other physicians on staff	1	2	3	4	5
e.	Comfort of the physical surroundings	1	2	3	4	5
f.	Hospital staff's concern for your well being	1	2	3	4	5
g.	Administration of drugs and medications	1	2	3	4	5
h.	Admitting procedures	1	2	3	4	5
i.	Discharging procedures	1	2	3	4	5
j.	Parking for visitors	1	2	3	4	5
k.	Quality of food	1	2	3	4	5
l.	Concern for relatives who visit or call	1	2	3	4	5
m.	Quality of instructions for care after discharge	1	2	3	4	5
n.	Costs	1	2	3	4	5

7. Which hospital would you go to for each of the following services or treatments (please identify):
   a. Heart treatment _____
   b. Delivery and care of babies _____
   c. Cancer treatment _____
   d. Mental health services _____
   e. Chemical dependency services _____
   f. General surgery _____
   g. Pediatric care _____
   h. General medicine _____
   i. Emergency care _____
   j. Surgery not requiring an overnight stay _____
   k. Orthopedic (bone) surgery _____
   l. Ear, nose, and throat surgery _____
   m. Gynecological surgery _____
   n. Neurological problems (diseases of the brain and nervous system) _____
   o. Ophthalmological (eye) surgery _____
   p. Urology problems _____

8. How long has it been since you or someone else in your family visited a hospital emergency department for treatment or examination?
   a. Less than   b. Six months   c. One to two   d. Two to five
      six months   to a year   years   years
   e. More than   f. Never
      five years

9. Which hospital's emergency department did you go to?

   _____

10. Why did you select that hospital for your emergency department services?
   a. Good   b. Recommended   c. Ambulance
      location   by doctor   took me/
                                               them

   d. Referred by   e. Had been   f. My doctor
      emergency   there   practices there
      phone   before
      number

   g. Other (please specify): _____

11. How would you rate the quality of care you received as an emergency patient?

		Excellent	Good	Fair	Poor	Do Not Know
a.	Courtesy of staff	1	2	3	4	5
b.	Courtesy of physicians	1	2	3	4	5
c.	Quality of medical treatment	1	2	3	4	5
d.	Laboratory/ x-ray services	1	2	3	4	5
e.	Patient instruction upon discharge	1	2	3	4	5
f.	Concern for patient's condition	1	2	3	4	5
g.	Quality of nursing care	1	2	3	4	5
h.	Speed of service/ treatment	1	2	3	4	5
i.	Concern for relatives of patients	1	2	3	4	5
j.	Privacy of visit	1	2	3	4	5
k.	Reception by admitting staff	1	2	3	4	5
l.	Costs	1	2	3	4	5

Please comment: _____

_____

12. How would you rate the following health care services in your immediate community? (Circle a response for each service.)

		Excellent	Good	Fair	Poor	Do Not Know
a.	Health promotion and education	1	2	3	4	5
b.	Home health care	1	2	3	4	5
c.	Ambulance	1	2	3	4	5
d.	Emergency room	1	2	3	4	5
e.	Counseling for emotional problems	1	2	3	4	5
f.	Up-to-date medical and hospital care	1	2	3	4	5
g.	Nursing homes	1	2	3	4	5
h.	Treatment of emergency and nonemergency alcohol and drug problems	1	2	3	4	5
i.	Number of family physicians	1	2	3	4	5
j.	HMO	1	2	3	4	5
k.	Number of physician specialists	1	2	3	4	5
l.	Services for the elderly	1	2	3	4	5
m.	Other	1	2	3	4	5

(please specify: _____)

n. Write in the letter from above that you think is the *most* in need of improvement. _____
Why? _____

o. Write in the letter from above that you think is the *second most* in need of improvement. _____
Why? _____

p. Write in the letter from above that you think is the *third most* in need of improvement. _____
Why? _____

13. How important to you are the following aspects of a hospital when you choose one? (Circle a response for each aspect.)

		Very Important	Somewhat Important	Not Important
a.	Located close to home	1	2	3
b.	Located close to work	1	2	3
c.	Cost	1	2	3
d.	Quality of food	1	2	3
e.	Cleanliness	1	2	3
f.	Quietness	1	2	3
g.	Appearance of the hospital building	1	2	3
h.	Friendliness of the employees	1	2	3
i.	Quality of nursing care	1	2	3
j.	Physicians who practice at the hospital	1	2	3
k.	Emergency department with a full-time physician	1	2	3
l.	Comfortable visitors' lounges	1	2	3
m.	Full-time spiritual and psychological support service	1	2	3
n.	Community health education programs	1	2	3
o.	Specific clinical services (obstetrics, pediatrics, neurology, and so forth)	1	2	3
p.	An understandable bill	1	2	3
q.	Other (please specify): _____	1	2	3

14. Do you or your family currently maintain a relationship with a physician who could be called your family physician?
    a. Yes   b. No

15. Would you change your family physician if you could find one more conveniently located?
    a. Yes   b. No   c. Do not know

16. Are there enough family physicians in your immediate community?
a. Yes   b. No

17. How many miles round trip do you travel to get to your family physician? _____ miles

18. Where is your physician's office or clinic located?

_____

19. How would you rate the following aspects of your physician's practice?

		Excellent	Good	Fair	Poor	Do Not Know
a.	Office location	1	2	3	4	5
b.	Office hours	1	2	3	4	5
c.	Physicians	1	2	3	4	5
d.	Nurses	1	2	3	4	5
e.	Courtesy of office staff	1	2	3	4	5
f.	Charges (fees)	1	2	3	4	5
g.	Quality of medical treatment	1	2	3	4	5
h.	Promptness of appointments	1	2	3	4	5
i.	Availability of appointments	1	2	3	4	5
j.	Availability of physician of your choice	1	2	3	4	5
k.	Concern for patient's condition	1	2	3	4	5
l.	Other (please specify): _____	1	2	3	4	5

20. How interested would you be in learning more about Medical Center, through an advertisement, regarding each of the following topics:

	Very Interested	Somewhat Interested	Not at all Interested
a. Range of services available	1	2	3
b. Concern for patient	1	2	3
c. Quality of hospital staff	1	2	3
d. Quality of medical staff	1	2	3
e. Facilities	1	2	3
f. Hospital costs and charges	1	2	3
g. Access	1	2	3

21. What is the best way for a hospital to reach you with information regarding services they have to offer you?

   a. Mail b. Television c. Radio d. Newspaper

   e. Personal f. Former g. Other (specify): _____
   physician patients

22. What is your experience with the Medical Center?_____
   a. I've been there and am generally satisfied because _____

   _____

   b. I've been there and am generally dissatisfied because_____

   _____

   c. I've never been there, but I have heard the following about the Medical Center:
   1. favorable comments 2. unfavorable comments 3. nothing

   Comments _____

23. Are you currently enrolled in an HMO (where the patient or family pays a group of physicians a monthly fee and they supply the health care services your family needs)?

   a. Yes b. No

   If yes, please specify:
   _____ Physicians' Health _____ Med Center
        Plan _____ HMO Minnesota
   _____ SHARE _____ Nicollet-Eitel
   _____ Group Health Plan _____ Coordinated Health
   _____ Ramsey Health Plan Care
   Other (please specify): _____

24. Which sex are you?   a. Male   b. Female

25. How old are you? _____

26. Are there children younger than 18 living with you?
    a. Yes   b. No

27. Are there persons older than 65 living with you?
    a. Yes   b. No

28. Do you occasionally care for (take to physician, or visit in a nursing home) someone who is older than 65?
    a. Yes   b. No

29. In which community do you live? _____
    How long? ___years

30. Which type of health insurance do you have? _____

31. If a new physician's office were opened in your community, what location would be ideal for you? _____

32. Additional comments: _____

    _____

    _____

THE MEDICAL CENTER THANKS YOU FOR YOUR HELP.

Appendix C

Monitoring Trends of the Medical Staff

Regardless of the level of sophistication at which an organization forecasts demand, prudent and effective planning dictate that health care organizations, particularly hospitals, carefully monitor the practice trends of their active medical staff. Not only is this critical in view of current payment policy (DRGs), but it also enables the health care organization to identify how such critical variables as patient mix and ancillary utilization will change in the future.

Most health care organizations have sophisticated computer equipment to enable effective monitoring of the practice style of the medical staff. Some critical variables include:
- Use of ancillary services
- Specialty
- Admitting profile, including types of patients and third-party payers
- Average length of stay
- Diagnosis
- Average charges

Another critical component to measure and monitor is information about the medical staff members themselves, such as their:
- Age
- Specialty
- Board certification
- Admissions record, that is, increase or decrease
- Office location
- Location of home

- Group size
- Admissions to (how many) other hospitals
- Hospital preference
- Contractual arrangements with HMOs

These data relate well to forecasting in many ways. For example, the forecasting hospital may note, by reviewing physician data, that all of the physicians in the organization's ear, nose, and throat medical staff complement are more than 60 years of age. The hospital will have to recruit such practitioners or that specialty will not represent a significant portion of patient mix in the future. Unless steps are taken to increase the number of these practitioners, the hospital's long-range forecast will have to reflect decreasing admissions in that specialty.

Another use of these data would be in the case of the "champion" admitter whose admissions have suddenly dropped off. Conducting an analysis might disclose that the physician is disgruntled about something and is admitting patients elsewhere. Further analysis might conclude that the physician has been ill or has substantially cut back office hours. Whether these findings are in or out of the health care organization's control will dictate the action to be taken. In any case, such information is critical to accurate planning and forecasting.

There are as many software packages as there are computers that will enable hospitals to monitor information about the medical staff. A good start would be to check with the hospital's hardware supplier or manufacturer to see whether any software packages exist that will assist in this critical aspect of demand forecasting.

Finally, physician input is vital to forecasting techniques that rely on judgment. Examples include the Delphi technique and the judgment worksheets (figures 8 and 9) discussed elsewhere in this book. Physicians are the hospital's best experts in the areas of changes in medical practice, trends in length of stay, and changing technology that will have an impact on ancillary demand and capital equipment needs. As such, the hospital cannot afford to neglect this vital source of information.

Appendix D

Excerpts from an Environmental Assessment

Introduction

The operating environment for hospitals continues to be volatile, with the marketplace undergoing a major transition to a more competitive model—an environment with new rules, new dynamics, and new markets. As the health care industry restructures, hospitals as the traditional providers are pressured to diversify into a wide variety of service roles. Strategy development in these new markets is hampered by a lack of understanding of the operating environment within each of these market segments. Health Central has therefore taken its environmental analysis a step further this year and produced a document that hospitals can use as a basis for their strategy development. The first section of this assessment examines major trends within the operating environment. The second section provides an analysis of the five emerging new markets for providers, and the third section, the strategic resources that Health Central believes will be critical to achieve success in the identified new markets.

Section 1: Major Trends within the Operating Environment

Change in the following areas have resulted in major trends within the operating environment:

The restructuring of the health care industry. Pressures in the environment are changing the underlying economics and structure of the health care industry. The marketplace is undergoing a major transition to a competitive model, with the new industry structure characterized by increasing merger activity and the entry of new providers into traditional markets and the hospital into less traditional emerging markets.

The recession of the U.S. economy. Despite declining inflation, the recessionary U.S. economy has a number of significant implications for the health care industry, including government cutbacks, the visibility of the hospital as an expensive resource, limited access to capital, reduced levels of insurance coverage, and increasingly discerning consumers.

Demographic change. The United States is experiencing a dramatic shift of population from the North and East to the South and West, and a growing proportion of elderly in the population.

Restrictive reimbursement. The hospital faces severe cutbacks in reimbursement and an increasingly complex payment environment. The changing reimbursement scene will have a profound effect on both the delivery of health services and the profitability of the industry. Government is cutting back through landmark legislation. Private payers and business are seeking cost reductions as cost-shifting continues. The marketplace will become more complex, more competitive, and more price sensitive. Hospitals must strive to maximize reimbursement under the new conditions.

Growth in alternative delivery systems. HMOs represent a significant component of the reimbursement matrix in many geographic areas in which the hospital operates. HMOs continue to increase in terms of number of plans and total enrollment. Private investment in HMOs is increasing, encouraged by the federal government. Preferred provider organizations are developing in various parts of the United States, representing a new form of selective contracting between payers and provider delivery systems.

Increasing consolidation within the health care industry. Investor-owned hospital management companies continue to experience significant growth; investment analysts vary in their projections of further growth that will result from the increasingly restrictive operating environment. The growth of multihospital systems continues, with changes in the way in which hospitals affiliate with systems.

Section 2: New Markets for Health

The trends described in section 1 are creating a restructured operating environment for hospitals and other health care providers: an environment with new rules, new dynamics, and new markets.

Noninstitutional services. Hospitals must increasingly look outside their four walls to provide services and pursue new sources of revenue, through both patient-related and nonpatient-related products. The following forces are creating market growth:
- Need for diversification
- Strong political and economic incentives to minimize use of costly inpatient services
- The competitive marketplace
- Changing habits and expectations of the health consumer
- Growth of ambulatory services outside the hospital environment
- Technology

The scope and nature of the market are as follows:
- Markets for noninstitutional services fall into both patient-related and nonpatient-related.
- Patient-related markets cover the range of provisions from ambulatory surgery centers through home and hospice care to nurse-supported hotel rooms and wellness centers.
- Nonpatient-related markets range from shared management services to real estate and contract management.
- Competing providers in both marketplaces are low-cost providers, specialty firms, major nonhealth corporations, and other hospitals.

The following success factors are critical for market entry:
- Decide whether to "buy or build."
- Be prepared for financial losses during the first years of operation.
- Explore alternative legal and financial structures for the development of new service offerings.
- Use market research and carefully developed marketing programs.
- Ensure that the necessary human and capital resources are available.

New physician partnerships. The physician marketplace is being restructured. Physicians, like hospitals, are anxious to maintain both patient volumes and fees. Many opportunities exist in the competitive environment for partnerships between hospitals and physicans or physician groups.

The following forces are creating market growth:
- Physician supply
- Changing practice patterns

- Changing attitudes toward physicians

The scope and nature of the market includes the following potential services and facilities for partnerships:

- Administrative services
- Clinical hospital-based services
- Medical office buildings
- High-technology diagnosis equipment
- Primary and convenience care centers
- Ambulatory surgery and emergicenters
- Occupational health and industrial clinics
- PPOs and HMOs
- Closed staff

The following relationships with physicians are possible:

- Informal
- Purchased physician services
- Market or lease services to physicians
- Limited partnerships
- General partnerships
- Corporation

The following are critical factors for market entry:

- Willingness to take a leadership position
- A clear understanding of the marketplace, motivations among local physicians, and alternative legal and financial structures
- A willingness to act and take risks
- Capital and human resources
- Aggressive marketing programs

The elderly. Services to the elderly are becoming attractive and necessary markets for hospitals to pursue. Diversification of hospital programs and collaboration with other organizations are methods being used to provide for the needs of the elderly.

The following forces are creating market growth:

- Growth in the numbers of elderly
- Consumer demands
- Fragmented delivery and financing systems

The scope and nature of the market are as follows:

- The market is significantly different from traditional hospital markets, representing a diversity of need.
- Services require a shift from the medical model and coordination with the traditional network of aging services.
- The profile of potential services ranges from research and education through housing and transportation to home care.

- A variety of capital financing sources are available to aid hospitals in developing services for the elderly.

The following success factors are critical for market entry:

- Develop an in-depth understanding of the elderly population and its diverse market segments.
- Be willing to experiment, and explore creative financing opportunities.
- Attract and retain specialized human resources.
- Have a strong level of commitment from board, medical staff, and CEO to develop and sustain services for the elderly.
- Develop credibility and relationships with existing agencies in the field of aging services.

Employers. Employers are becoming increasingly concerned with the drastic increase in their employee health care costs and with their perceived lack of control over these costs. They are taking action as they see little from the government or health care industry. Existing health care providers have the necessary resources to provide programs to meet the needs of this significant market segment.

The following forces are creating market growth:

- Escalating health care costs
- Increasing interest in employee wellness and lifestyle
- Provider reaction to the competitive marketplace, with incentives to maintain patient volume
- Actions taken by employers, such as self-insurance, business coalitions, and private utilization review

The scope and nature of the market are as follows:

- Employers have a range of needs that can be met by health care providers, ranging from the need to reduce overall health costs through occupational health to the identification of low-cost providers.
- The potential response of health care organizations covers a broad spectrum of services, both clinical and administrative.

The following factors are critical for market entry:

- Thorough market research of needs and perceptions of the potential employers market
- The organizational ability to pull together a packaged product of real value to business
- Capital
- Specialized knowledge of business and industry practices, and human resources to support these programs

International markets. International market opportunities for American hospital management companies continue to expand, but must be approached with both caution and commitment.

The following forces are creating market growth:
- Demand for U.S. health care management expertise overseas
- Growth of the private sector of health care in both developed and developing countries
- U.S. government support for the export of health care services
- Individual company interests in expanding spheres of influence and potential profits

The scope and nature of the market are as follows:
- Market opportunities fall into two basic categories: short-term management/consulting contracts and long-term equity investment.
- Short-term contracts carry fewer risks and less capital need, the predominant market being made up of developing countries.
- Long-term investment has greater long-term profit potential, but carries greater risks and requires considerably more investment. Potential markets are economically stable countries with an impetus in the private sector.

The following factors are critical for market entry:
- In-depth knowledge of the economic, political, and cultural environment, and of the structure of the health sector in the host country
- A long-term commitment to business opportunities
- Rigorous feasibility analyses of potential projects
- Access to capital and high-quality personnel networks
- Maintenance of high-level government and community relations
- A commitment to train local host country personnel

Section 3: Areas of Strategic Resource Requirements

This section provides an analysis of five major areas of strategic resource requirements that the hospital must develop or have access to in order to compete effectively in the new markets identified in section 2.

Capital. Capital is the most critical strategic resource for hospitals and other health providers in the marketplace of the 1984s. Hospitals that want to diversify successfully must secure access to capital markets.

The following trends are occurring in hospital capital markets:
- Hospitals need capital for replacement and remodeling, funding of acquisitions, mergers and consolidations, diversification, and keeping pace with technology.
- Hospitals are being driven to the debt markets through declines in government funds, philanthropy, and their reduced equity positions.

- Capital markets are at the same time becoming increasingly inaccessible and multi-option.

The following initiatives should be undertaken to gain access to capital:

- Recognize the importance of capital to survival and the link between capital and bottom-line performance.
- Develop aggressive capital management strategies in the areas of forecasting, relationships with investment banking firms, refinancing, corporate reorganization, affiliation with multihospital systems, and the attraction of philanthropic support.

New organizational arrangements. Hospitals and health care organizations will need new organizational structures and arrangements to maximize revenues and position themselves competitively in the changing health care marketplace.

The following trends in organizational arrangements are occurring:

- Forces creating the need for restructuring include the new competitive marketplace, third-party reimbursement limitations, the increasing numbers of alternative health services options, and a diminishing capital and operational financial base.
- Hospitals are reorganizing for a number of reasons, the primary reason being reimbursement problems.
- Reorganized not-for-profit hospitals are forming new entities as taxable organizations. Taxable entities can enable and enhance the hospital's ability to compete and participate effectively in both new and traditional markets.

The following initiatives should be undertaken to develop new organizational arrangements:

- Develop a sound strategic plan providing direction to the new organizational configuration, and business plans for each new enterprise under consideration.
- Make sure restructuring offers significant benefits to the organization and is based on sound business advice.
- Ensure that appropriate capital and human resources are available to support the new, more complex enterprise.

Sophisticated management systems. Sophisticated management systems, systems dealing with both human and technical resources, are essential to the successful operation of the hospital in the changing marketplace. These management systems will be increasingly computer based.

The following trends in management systems are occurring:

- The increasingly complex operating environment demands for cost-effective production and increasing financial accountability,

the shift from an industrial to informational society, and rapid technological development are creating the need for sophisticated management systems.
- A wide range of management systems with emphasis on planning and productivity are now available to the hospital.
- Sophisticated management systems will be increasingly computer based.

The following initiatives should be undertaken to develop sophisticated management systems:
- Recognize that systems require significant financial investment and commitment from management and that they must be developed on an appropriate scale for the organization.
- Get expert advice on the evaluation and introduction of systems.
- Make sure the organization has the necessary human, financial, and technical resources to support the systems.
- Educate managers and users as to the goals, use, and application of the systems.

Technology. Technology is essential to the operation of the successful hospital in both clinical and management applications. The management of technology on an appropriate scale is a critical issue facing the hospital.

The following trends in technology are occurring:
- The technological development explosion continues to occur in both clinical and nonclinical areas.
- Constraints on technological acquisition include limited capital availability, equipment obsolescence, and reimbursement limits.

The following initiatives should be undertaken to gain access to technology:
- Carefully project capital requirements for new technology.
- Consider the need for and flexibility to upgrade new technology, product performance, manufacturer support, and projected financial return before purchase.
- Explore the potential of either sharing expensive technology with other providers or leasing equipment.
- Ensure adequately trained or retrained personnel are available to operate the technology.

Human resources management. Human resources represents a significant proportion of any health care organization's budget. Effective human resource management is essential in an environment demanding creativity and cost efficiency.

The following trends and forces are creating the need for improved human resources:

- The need for cost efficiency in a competitive environment
- Changes in both the U.S. and health industry labor force
- Proliferation of new technologies
- The need for recruitment of sophisticated management professionals
- Inadequate training of health care managers in human resources management

The following initiatives should be undertaken to develop human resources management:

- Recognize changing dynamics between management and employees, and become more responsive to employee needs.
- Develop productivity improvement strategies.
- Develop creative compensation packages for management personnel.
- Respond to the changing physician work force.
- Recruit skilled human resources professionals and new types of managers.

Bibliography

Articles

Armstrong, J. Scott. Economic forecasting and the science court. *Journal of Business*. 1978 Apr. 51:595.

Fetter, Robert B., and others. Case mix definition by diagnostic-related groups. *Medical Care*. 1980 Feb. 18(2, Supplement).

Fildes, Robert, and others. Forecasting in conditions of uncertainty. *Long Range Planning*. 1978 Aug. 2:29.

Fogler, H. R. A pattern recognition model for forecasting. *Management Science*. 1974 Apr. 20:1173.

Goldstone, L. Forecasting: unknowns and intangibles. *Health Social Services Journal*. 1980 Feb. 90:285.

Hall, W. K. Forecasting techniques for use in the corporate planning process. *Management Planning*. 1972 Nov.-Dec. 20:5.

Harrington, Michael B. Forecasting areawide demand for health care services: a critical review of major techniques and their applications. *Inquiry*. 1977 Sept. Vol. 14.

Higgins, J. C., and Romano, O. Social forecasting: an integral part of corporate planning? *Long Range Planning*. 1980 Apr. 13:82.

Hoyle, R. S. Capital budgeting models and planning: an evolutionary challenge. *Management Planning*. 1978 Nov.-Dec. 27:24.

Lebell, D., and Krasner, O. J. Selecting environmental forecasting techniques from business planning requirements. *Academic Management Review.* 1977 July. 2:373.

Linneman, R. E., and Klein, H. E. The use of multiple scenarios by U.S. industrial companies. *Long Range Planning.* 1979 Feb. 12:83.

Macnulty, C., and Macnulty, R. Scenario development for corporate planning. *Futures.* 1977 Apr. 9:128.

Newhouse, J. P. Forecasting demand for medical care for the purpose of planning health services. Report of the Rand Corporation, 1974.

Redmond, W. H. Values in forecasting and planning. *Long Range Planning.* 1978 June. 11:22.

Thurston, P. H. Make TF serve corporate planning. *Harvard Business Review.* 1971 Sept.-Oct. 49:98.

Walker, Lawrence R., and Greenawald, Edward, R. Two simple, accurate forecasting models. *Hospital Financial Management.* 1978 Mar. Page 16.

Walsh, D. C., and Bickinell, W. J. Forecasting the need for hospital beds: a quantitative methodology. *Public Health Report.* 1977 May-June. 92:199.

Whittle, J. Problems of corporate forecasting. *Accountancy.* 1978 Apr. 89:105.

Books

Armstrong, J. Scott. *Long Range Forecasting: From Crystal Ball to Computer.* New York City: John Wiley and Sons, Inc., 1978.

Ascher, William. *Forecasting: An Appraisal for Policy Makers and Planners.* Baltimore: Johns Hopkins Press, 1978.

Griffith, J. R. *Quantitative Techniques for Hospital Planning and Control.* Lexington, MA: Lexington Books, 1972.

MacStravic, Robin Scott. *Forecasting Use of Health Services: A Provider's Guide.* Rockville, MD: Aspen Systems Corp., 1984.

Wheelwright, S. C., and Makridakis, Spyros. *Forecasting Methods for Management.* 2nd ed. New York City: John Wiley and Sons, Inc., 1977.